D0349888

JAN   2014

Fit at Last

Fit at Last

LOOK AND FEEL BETTER
ONCE AND FOR ALL

Ken Blanchard

Tim Kearin

BK

Berrett–Koehler Publishers, Inc.
San Francisco
a BK Life book

Berrett-Koehler Publishers, Inc.
235 Montgomery Street, Suite 650
San Francisco, CA 94104-2916
Tel: (415) 288-0260   Fax: (415) 362-2512   www.bkconnection.com

Ordering Information
Quantity sales. Special discounts are available on quantity purchases by corporations, associations, and others. For details, contact the "Special Sales Department" at the Berrett-Koehler address above.
Individual sales. Berrett-Koehler publications are available through most bookstores. They can also be ordered directly from Berrett-Koehler: Tel: (800) 929-2929; Fax: (802) 864-7626; www.bkconnection.com
Orders for college textbook/course adoption use. Please contact Berrett-Koehler: Tel: (800) 929-2929; Fax: (802) 864-7626.
Orders by U.S. trade bookstores and wholesalers. Please contact Ingram Publisher Services, Tel: (800) 509-4887; Fax: (800) 838-1149; E-mail: customer. service@ingrampublisherservices.com; or visit www.ingrampublisherservices.com/ Ordering for details about electronic ordering.

Production Management: Michael Bass Associates
Cover Design: Irene Morris

Berrett-Koehler and the BK logo are registered trademarks of Berrett-Koehler Publishers, Inc.

SLII® is a registered trademark of The Ken Blanchard Companies.

This book contains the opinions and ideas of its authors, who are not medical professionals. The contents are strictly for informational and entertainment purposes and are not a substitute for medical advice. Always consult a qualified healthcare professional before you begin any exercise or nutrition program or if you have questions about your health.

Printed in the United States of America

Berrett-Koehler books are printed on long-lasting acid-free paper. When it is available, we choose paper that has been manufactured by environmentally responsible processes. These may include using trees grown in sustainable forests, incorporating recycled paper, minimizing chlorine in bleaching, or recycling the energy produced at the paper mill.

Library of Congress Cataloging-in-Publication Data

Blanchard, Kenneth H.
    Fit at last : look and feel better once and for all / Ken Blanchard, Tim Kearin.
        pages cm.
    ISBN 978-1-62656-060-4 (hardback)
    1. Physical fitness. I. Kearin, Timothy. II. Title.
    GV481.B489 2014
    613.7—dc23   2013038756

First Edition
18 17 16 15 14 • 10 9 8 7 6 5 4 3 2 1

*We dedicate this book to all of you who struggle
to be as healthy as possible but run into occasional
trouble behaving on your good intentions.*

Contents

Introduction:
Keeping Your Commitment
to Your Commitment

Have you ever made New Year's resolutions that you didn't keep? My experience is that all of us have had good intentions to do things over the years, yet we didn't follow through. We usually start out enthusiastic about the change, and then after a while our enthusiasm goes by the wayside. Why is that?

It's my contention that the old adage "The road to nowhere is paved with good intentions" is probably more true than we want to admit. My friend and colleague Art Turock, author of many books—including a classic on health and fitness entitled *Getting Physical*—argues that the problem stems from the difference between *interest* and *commitment*. For example, when *interested* exercisers who have started a jogging or walking program wake up and find it is raining outside, they lie back down and say to themselves, "I think I'll exercise tomorrow." However, when *committed* exercisers wake up and find it's raining, they get out of bed and say to themselves, "I think I'll exercise inside today." People who are *interested* in doing something will do it if all goes as planned—but give them a hiccup or two and they don't follow through. People who are *committed*

1

to do something will continue to do it, no matter what. In other words:

They keep their commitment to their commitment.

So let's get real. What have you been wanting to do for a long time but just haven't been able to accomplish? Maybe it has to do with fitness—physical activity and weight control—which I had procrastinated about for a long time. Or perhaps it's more about improving yourself on the inside or other aspects of a healthy lifestyle, and you'd like to focus on becoming more resilient, creative, generous, or empathetic. You might want to push yourself to improve your communication skills, get organized, do volunteer work, or spend more time with your family. Maybe you've been making excuses for years instead of sitting down and writing that novel or learning to speak French. This book may help you move from being *interested* in doing it to being *committed* to doing it—*no matter what*.

Beginning January 1, 2011, the Boomer generation began turning 65 at the rate of 10,000 per day. This rate will continue for 19 years. Research shows that many in this generation intend not to retire but to continue to work and play hard. Many others can't afford to retire because of unfortunate circumstances or poor retirement planning. Either way, it is imperative that adults maintain their optimal health and fitness no matter what their age.

Every year in January following a New Year's resolution, thousands of people begin an exercise program with the idea that it will change their lives forever. By the end of March, about 90 percent of those who started are no longer participating—not because they have changed their minds about the importance of exercise, but because exercise is hard work and they are not seeing the immediate results they had hoped for. Whatever the reason, they don't follow through.

This book follows my journey from interest to commitment about my fitness. The western heroic legend of the lone wolf who succeeds at lofty goals based solely on strength of will and sharp wit is strong with many people. This "John Wayne myth" isn't dead—it's just not effective. As you'll learn, I could not keep my commitment to an effective fitness plan alone. I needed help. That help came from my coauthor Tim Kearin, a health and fitness coach who had been patient with me for many years.

Each year Tim listened to me make an announcement about what I was going to do about my fitness that year, and then he watched me not keep my commitment. Year after year we went through the same routine: Tim would receive a call from me early in the year—usually February, since I didn't want to join the New Year's resolution crowd—to begin a fitness program. I would get underway with enthusiasm, but after a month or so I would gradually become too busy to keep my commitment to my commitment. The process would start again at the beginning of the next year.

So follow along and see how Tim and I broke this ineffective cycle. I know *Fit at Last* will help you behave on your good intentions and keep your commitment to your commitment, no matter what issue you are working on.

Ken Blanchard
Coauthor, *The One Minute Manager*®

A Joint Commitment

Ken's Story

Think about an exciting story. Doesn't it always have an interesting character who wants to make something important happen in their life, but first has to overcome conflict to accomplish the goal? Well, the interesting character in this story is me. What I want to accomplish that is important is to become fit again so I will feel better and live longer. To do that, I have to overcome conflict—my past patterns of behavior and how I dealt with the ups and downs of life.

As I tell you my story, I'm probably going to tell you more about the ups and downs of my life than you want to hear. Why? I've found that a lot of people think that because I've been fairly successful in my life, everything has gone along smoothly and all the breaks went my way. This was not always the case.

I was born in 1939 and grew up in New Rochelle, New York. My mom was a very nurturing person. Unfortunately, one of the ways she nurtured us best was by feeding us. If we were happy, we ate. If we were sad, we ate. If we were worried, we ate. Whatever

5

happened, we ate. One of the ways Mom self-actualized was through the food she gave my father, my sister, and me. As I grew up, I used to fantasize about being locked in our local Jewish delicatessen overnight. I can smell a piece of cheesecake a mile away.

Given that reality, you might ask—with the pattern of eating I got from my mother and my love of cheesecake— why I wasn't obese. Actually, the first 25 years of my life, even though my mom fed us well, I was pretty fit and exercised a lot. But it didn't start out that way.

I was born with flat feet. In those days, the belief was that kids with flat feet wouldn't be able to live normal lives in terms of exercise and activity, because they would get tired and need to rest. My mother accepted that belief and continually was watching that I didn't overdo things. That worked until I was six years old, when my dad put a basket in our basement and I fell in love with basketball. It became my passion. I would shoot by the hour. I led our elementary team to the city championship, played in a number of different leagues in junior high school, broke the junior varsity scoring record my sophomore year in high school, and was cocaptain of our league champion high school team my senior year. What did that mean in terms of my fitness? I was in good shape. I used to run cross-country in the fall to get ready for basketball season. So fitness and weight control were not a problem the first 18 years of my life.

When it came to choosing a college, I decided to go to Cornell University in Ithaca, New York. I tried out for the freshman basketball team there and made the squad, but since I had not been recruited by Sam McNeill, the coach, he seldom played me. I remember one night when we were playing Auburn Community College in a small band-box gym. They played a two-one-two zone defense that made it difficult to score except from the outside—my specialty. Our starting team was struggling so I got off the bench, kneeled by Coach McNeill, and said, "Put me in, Coach. I could break up this zone in my sleep. After all, I have the hottest hands in the country." He laughed and started calling me "Hot Hands" but still didn't play me much, although we became good friends.

Rather than realizing the potential of gathering more splinters on the bench, I decided not to go out for the team my sophomore year and instead became a cheerleader. You might think that would have been good for me, with all the gymnastics. Wrong. In those days, cheerleaders didn't do gymnastics—and since we were the only co-ed school in the Ivy League, we weren't allowed to have women cheerleaders. The only criteria for being a cheerleader was (1) you had to drink and (2) you had to know a lot of people. I qualified on both counts, but it didn't do my fitness any good.

During my senior year at Cornell, Coach McNeill was promoted to varsity coach. He asked me to help coach the freshman team because we had kept in touch and he knew I understood the game. This was a thrill for me and got me reenergized about basketball.

The summer after my graduation in 1961, Margie and I began to date. Our romance blossomed that fall as I continued my studies at Colgate University, where I began a master's degree program in sociology while Margie was finishing her senior year at Cornell.

In June 1962 after I had completed my first year at Colgate, Margie and I got married. We spent the summer honeymooning at a well-known canoe tripping camp in Algonquin

Park on Canoe Lake in Ontario, Canada. To get a snack, you had to walk uphill five miles or canoe three miles. So I returned to Colgate in probably the best shape of my life, weighing 167.

That didn't last for long, though—Margie was a great cook, and working on my master's thesis required long hours sitting in the library. My basketball coaching did help prevent a complete downward spiral, as I was asked to work with the freshman team at Colgate for the 1962–63 season.

When I was nearing completion of my master's program, I told my Student Personnel Administration mentors at Cornell that I was ready to become a dean. They suggested it would be better if I first got my doctoral degree. Through a former professor at Cornell, I was accepted into the doctoral program in educational administration there. That began my three-year Ph.D. journey.

Basketball was still a major interest, so as a player-coach I organized a team that was sponsored by Hal's Delicatessen in downtown Ithaca. We competed all over central New York against other town teams made up of former high school and college basketball players. We even got to play the Cornell freshman team as the preliminary game to Senator Bill Bradley and his Princeton Tigers' last visit to Cornell in 1964. They opened the doors for the game at 6:00, and by 6:30 they had the largest crowd in the history of Cornell: over 10,000 people poured into our arena. So all those fans had to watch our preliminary game, which we won.

While I continued to play ball, I didn't go at it with the vigor that I had when I was younger, and I began to gain weight. Why? With Hal's Delicatessen as the sponsor of our team, my fantasy of being locked overnight in a deli unfortunately began to become a reality. Hal's had the best cheesecake imaginable.

One thing I was proud of, though, was that I put my head down and made it through the doctoral program, including my dissertation. While I was doing that, Margie completed her master's degree in speech pathology—her undergraduate major—and gave birth to our son, Scott, in August 1965.

When I was working on my dissertation our last year in Ithaca, I didn't have time to coach or play for Hal's Delicatessen team and started to get a little pudgy. Even though I didn't play for the team, I still visited Hal's on a regular basis to make sure all was well.

My pudginess continued as I finally entered the world of work. In the fall of 1966 after nine years of college, Margie (pregnant with Debbie), Scott, and I all headed to Ohio University where I had landed a job as assistant to Harry Evarts, dean of the School of Business Administration.

Let me take an important detour from discussing my fitness journey. When I joined Dean Evarts's staff, he asked me to teach a course in the management department. I had never thought about teaching—all of my professors in graduate school had said if I wanted to work at a university, I needed to be an administrator because I couldn't write. As a faculty member, if you didn't write, it was career damaging. The rule was "publish or perish."

Harry said he didn't care about all of that. All he knew was that he wanted all of his deans to teach a course so they were really in tune with the students. Paul Hersey had just arrived on campus as the chairman of the management department. Harry put me in his department and Hersey gave me a course to teach. After teaching for a couple of weeks, I came home and said to Margie, "This is what I ought to be doing. Teaching is fun."

Margie was quick to respond, "But what about the writing?"

I said, "I don't know, but we'll figure something out."

That fall I heard that Hersey taught a tremendous leadership course, so I came up to him in a hallway in December 1966 and said, "Paul, I understand you teach a great leadership course. Could I sit in next semester?"

Hersey said, "Nobody audits my course. If you want to take it for credit, you're welcome." And he walked away. I thought that was something because I had a Ph.D. and he didn't! *And he wants me to take his course?*

I went home and told Margie about the conversation. She said, "Is he any good?"

I said, "He's supposed to be fabulous."

"Then why don't you get your ego out of the way and take his course?"

So I took the course, wrote all the papers, and found it to be a great experience.

In June 1967 after the course had ended, Hersey came to my office and sat down. He said, "Ken, I've been teaching leadership for 10 years now and I think I'm better than anybody. But I can't write and they want me to write a textbook. I'm a nervous wreck. I've been looking for a good writer like you. Would you write it with me?"

I almost laughed out loud when he said "a good writer like you."

Why not? I thought. *We ought to be a good team. He can't write and I'm not supposed to, so let's do it.*

That's exactly what we did. We wrote a textbook entitled *Management of Organizational Behavior: Utilizing Human Resources*. It recently came out in its 10th edition, and I think it sells more today than it did in the 1960s.

When the book was published, I went to Dean Evarts and said, "I quit."

He said, "You can't quit because I was going to fire you. You're a lousy administrator!"—which I was. We agreed it was a photo finish between him firing me and me quitting. But that launched my career as a teacher and writer at age 30, with a few bumps along the way.

Why did I take a detour to tell you all this? A lot of people think that when you are successful, it means you had a plan when you were young, set your eyes on the target, and just kept moving toward it over the years. I haven't found that to be true. In fact, John Lennon said it well: "Life is what happens to you while you're busy making other plans." My ups and downs in life were not planned but were an important part of my journey.

How was my fitness at that time? Although Paul Hersey and I played in a city basketball league together, I wasn't in great shape. Working on the textbook was more demanding than working on my doctoral dissertation.

It was during that period I joined Weight Watchers for the first time to get some support for eating properly and losing weight. It helped, too, until Margie and the kids and I moved to Amherst, Massachusetts, in 1970. I was asked to play a major role in the educational administration department at the University of Massachusetts as well as work with school systems along the East Coast. Those activities, plus writing and teaching, sidetracked my fitness program again as I regained the weight I had lost and then some. I soon found myself hovering around 210 pounds. That wasn't good, to say the least, since when I was playing basketball I never tipped the scale over 175.

Discouraged, I wondered if I'd ever get in shape again. But finally, in 1974, I got serious, rejoined Weight Watchers, and got my weight back down under 190.

In spring 1976, all of Margie's and my hard work paid off. She earned her Ph.D. in communications, and I was promoted to full professor and given a one-year sabbatical leave, which we took in San Diego, California. We found San Diego to be a very healthy, exercise-friendly environment. I started jogging with Margie, even ran several 10K races, and kept myself in pretty good shape. Realizing that "summer in Massachusetts is two weeks of bad skating" and that San Diego probably has the best weather on the planet, it was not hard for us to decide to stay put and not return to Amherst at the end of the year. We began working with Paul Hersey, who had also moved to San Diego to launch the Center for Leadership Studies.

In 1979, Margie and I decided to start our own company. That turned out to be quite a year. My dad passed away in February, Margie got spinal meningitis that summer, my sister Sandy died in October, and Alan Raffe, a local CEO who had helped us start our company, was killed in an airplane accident in December. I'll never forget holding Margie on New Year's Eve as we hoped we would safely enter the next year.

The year 1980 did end up being a special year. In November, Margie and I met Spencer Johnson at a cocktail party. He was a children's book writer. He had coauthored, with his former wife, Ann, a series of kids' books called ValueTales. Margie met Spencer first, hand-carried him over to me, and said, "You two should write a children's book for managers. They won't read anything else." With that, *The One Minute*

Manager® was born. We signed a publishing contract with William Morrow in January 1982, and the book was launched on NBC's *Today* show on Labor Day that year. The book went on the *New York Times* best-seller list the next week and stayed there continually for a few years.

Prior to the instant success of the book, I had maintained a good exercise and eating program and was feeling proud of myself. Then suddenly the phone was ringing off the hook, and I was traveling around the world spreading "the word." My fitness program took a dive once more as I did not watch my eating habits, did little exercise, and began bulking up again. This motivated me in 1985 to write *The One Minute Manager Gets Fit* with Margie and our longtime friend Dee Edington, who was the director of the Fitness Research Center as well as professor and director of the Division of Physical Education at the University of Michigan in Ann Arbor.

During the writing of the book, with help from Dee and prodding from Margie, I got myself back in good shape. My weight was under control and I was exercising regularly. We even held a wellness seminar for top managers at Callaway Gardens in Georgia. That's when I first met Tim Kearin. He was working at the nearby Hughston Clinic as their fitness director. Tim was recommended by the president of Callaway Gardens, Hal Northrup, to do the fitness evaluations and consultations for our program there.

I immediately connected with Tim, not only as a professional but also as a human being. In fact, Margie and I were key encouragers in convincing Tim and his wife, Sharon, to move to San Diego the following year. But even after the inspiration of *The One Minute Manager Gets Fit* and our Georgia seminar, when Dee went back to his research and Margie decided to stop bugging me, I gradually gained weight again and stopped my regular exercising.

You might be saying, *Come on, Blanchard. I'm sick of hearing about this yo-yo weight and exercise thing with you. You write about motivation, you speak about motivation, and you even wrote a book about fitness. Why couldn't you keep your commitment to your commitment and keep on going with your fitness journey?*

My first response is a defensive one. "So who are you, Mr. or Ms. Perfect? Everything you say you'll do, you do? Give me a break. How many New Year's resolutions have you broken? If you can't think of any, you probably lie about other things, too."

My saner intellectual response is that there are three levels to change.

1. *Knowledge*—this is the easiest thing to change. All you have to do is listen to someone or read a book about something and you'll have new knowledge.
2. *Attitudinal*—this is more difficult to change than gaining knowledge. Why? Because attitude is an emotionally charged bit of knowledge. Now you feel either positive or negative about something you know.
3. *Behavioral*—this is the toughest thing to change, because you have to *do* something. I don't know a smoker alive today who doesn't know, at a knowledge level, that smoking is not good for them. Most smokers also have a positive attitude toward giving it up. But try it behaviorally if it's been a longtime habit—it's not easy. The same goes for me in curbing my childhood eating patterns and maintaining a good exercise program.

My longtime friend and colleague Fred Finch put it well when I told him about my fitness journey. I said, "I just need to get better organized."

Fred was quick to reply. "Ken, you're the most organized person I have ever met *when you want to do something.*"

I knew Fred was right. At the knowledge and attitudinal levels I was ready to make a change, but not at the behavioral level—at least not completely. I would think about it at the beginning of every new year and would call Tim to start a workout program. But then, as usual, I'd get too busy and go on the road, and the workout program would fall by the wayside. This was discouraging, to say the least. Tim would encourage me to keep going, but after a while he would get discouraged, too, and move on to greener pastures—clients who were committed to a regular fitness program. I would rejoin Weight Watchers several more times and start going to the meetings, but then I would let my membership lapse and let that go, too. I felt frustrated that I was only *interested* in being fit, but somehow not *committed* to it.

PRINCIPLE 1
Have Compelling Reasons and a Purpose

Having compelling reasons and a purpose is what motivates you toward goal accomplishment. It's something to serve. Goals are to be accomplished; reasons and purpose are to be served. It became clear to me, if I was going to keep my commitment to my commitment, I needed some compelling reasons. Then, lo and behold, reasons started coming at me fast and furious.

First, when I turned 65 a few years ago, I was talking on the phone to Zig Ziglar, the great motivational expert who passed away late in 2012. He had invited Margie and me to the 59th anniversary of his 21st birthday. I asked him, "Zig, are you going to retire?" He was quick to reply, "There is no mention of retirement in the Bible. Except for Jesus, Mary, Joseph, David, and a few others, no one under 80 made an impact. As a result . . .

"I'm not retiring—I'm refiring!"

That really resonated with me. I decided to follow Zig's lead and *refire,* not retire. To that end, I had to get myself back in shape so I could walk easily through airports and stand in front of groups and inspire them to lead at a higher level.

Over the next several years I had both hips replaced, and it was suggested that I have a total knee replacement as well. My primary physician, Dr. Lee Rice—who used to be the team physician for the San Diego Chargers—indicated that I might avoid this surgery with strength training and weight loss. Since I had heard that rehab from knee operations was much tougher than from hip surgery, my attitude started to change. Then two other events added to this motivation.

My son Scott and I flew to London to work with some of our clients. He noticed that I was not only gimping around and looking a lot like Quasimodo from *The Hunchback of Notre Dame,* but also huffing and puffing whenever we had to walk anywhere. He finally lost it and said to me, "Dad, I've heard you kid around and say to Mom that when a tour bus unloads passengers at a hotel in Hawaii, 35 women will get off the bus and only 5 men, because the rest of the guys are dead. And you always say that your goal is to be one of those 5 guys. What are you doing about it? I know you don't want to leave Mom a widow. You talk about wanting to be at the college graduations of your grandsons Kurtis, Kyle, and Alec. You're going to have to hang around at least another 15 years. What are you doing about it?"

I didn't really have a good answer. I knew that my lack of focus on my health and fitness just wasn't making sense. After all, if I didn't take care of myself, I might miss out not only on aging with my best friend Margie, but also on watching our kids Scott and Debbie get their letters from AARP, seeing my grandkids grow up, and being with my best four-legged friend.

Four-legged friend?

In November 2008, three weeks before I had my first hip replacement operation, we decided to get a new puppy. We named her Joy, because a wonderful business friend of mine, Fred Smith, often said:

"Real joy in life is when you get in the act of forgetfulness about yourself."

Dogs, particularly puppies, help you do that.

Joy is a miniature "golden doodle"—a cross between a golden retriever and a poodle. We were told that fully grown she would be between 15 and 20 pounds. She's all black and doesn't look anything like a golden retriever, but she loves to retrieve, which is not a normal behavior for a poodle.

After my operation I was home for five or six weeks rehabbing, and Joy and I really bonded. When I would go out to do an errand or go to the office, she would follow me to the door. The minute I got home, opened the door to the garage, and came into the house, she would come racing down the hall toward me and jump into my arms.

When we got Joy, I was just turning 70. Knowing that little dogs can last 15 years or more, I decided I needed to be in good health until my mid-80s so not only would I be around for Margie, my kids, and grandkids, but this little dog would never run down the hall without finding me there. I know this seems a little strange because most people who love dogs are more concerned about losing their dog than having their dog lose them. But as you probably have guessed by now, I don't always think like other people.

Even though I was frustrated about not having been able to stick to a fitness program because of past failures, I now had all kinds of reasons that motivated me to get serious and take on this project with Tim, who had tried to help me with my periodic fitness commitments over the past 25 years. I still felt Tim had the personal power—he's one of my favorite people—and the most expertise to help me achieve my goals. I knew I was no John Wayne type when it came to my own fitness.

This book follows Tim's and my journey through a one-year fitness program where, finally, I realized that if I were going to become fit, I would need to behave on my good intentions *for myself* rather than because others close to me said I should do it—or wagged their tails.

Even though it might have taken several decades for Tim and me to get to this point together, I'm excited about our adventure. I hope that by our sharing it with you, you'll be inspired to keep your commitment to your commitment to do something that will improve your life, too.

FOOD FOR THOUGHT

What have you been wanting to do for a long time but haven't yet been able to accomplish?

On a scale of 1 to 10, with 1 being dreadful and 10 being excellent, how would you rate your current fitness level?

What New Year's resolutions have you made in the past that you didn't keep? What happened? What can you do to ensure this won't happen again?

How many compelling reasons can you think of for improving your fitness level?

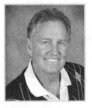

Tim's Story

My interest in making my body into a better-functioning machine began when I was 13 years old. At that time, I remember seeing advertisements in the back of magazines that would show a picture of Charles Atlas, one of the early musclemen. The first part of the ad showed a bully kicking sand in the face of a skinny boy at the beach and walking away with his bikini-clad girlfriend. The idea behind the Atlas program was to develop a strong, muscular body and win the girl back. This also tells you that I have been around long enough to be on the leading edge of the Boomer generation.

I began doing my own program of push-ups, pull-ups, and sit-ups. By age 14, my weight training program had progressed to barbells and dumbbells. That, along with pubertal hormones, allowed me to begin developing muscles. While I didn't go to the beach looking for bullies, I did enjoy that people began noticing my muscular shape. When I began high school, I was quickly recruited to play football. I was a hard-hitting, good blocking lineman but realized my muscles alone did not make me a better player. I soon realized that I needed to eat smarter and develop cardiovascular fitness.

What happened next would begin my inspiration for a lifetime of fitness. I was bench-pressing 400 pounds and had many world-class weight lifters suggest that if I took steroid supplements I could get bigger and stronger than I already was. While few sports administrations did any kind of testing for supplements, the only way you could get steroids was on the black market. As an uninformed, impressionable high school kid, I began my search. My first stop was my neighbor's house. My best friend's dad was Chuck Coker, a highly recognized fitness authority and co-inventor of the Universal Gym, one of the first multiple-station strength training machines. Chuck lectured me about all of the negative effects of steroid use. His talk scared me so much that I became an activist against steroid supplements. I worked summers doing deliveries and demonstrations on the Universal Gym. I learned a great deal about strength training from Chuck, and he inspired me to a lifetime career in the fitness industry.

I went to the University of Arizona on an athletic scholarship and, following graduation, began a military career. My fitness prowess as a junior officer led to my selection to attend graduate school at Indiana University and go on to the United States Military Academy. While working in the physical education department, I became involved in strength training research under Arthur Jones, founder of Nautilus Equipment, Inc. I later became one of the United States Military Academy's early strength and conditioning coaches. I directed the conditioning programs for more than 15 intercollegiate athletic teams. West Point was synonymous with fitness, but it was very challenging to develop muscle mass on athletes who got inadequate sleep because of the rigorous schedule the cadets were required to keep. One of the main purposes of a good conditioning program is to prevent injury, so I became very involved with athletic rehabilitation.

After seven years at the military academy, I accepted a job at the Hughston Clinic in Georgia as director of cardiac rehab, back fitness, executive fitness testing, and adult fitness. As Ken mentioned, I was selected to run fitness evaluations and consultations for the executive wellness seminar that he, Margie, and Dee Edington were holding for top industry managers at Callaway Gardens, based on their book *The One Minute Manager Gets Fit*. That introduction began what would be a 25-year friendship and fitness relationship with Ken.

In 1986, I moved my family to San Diego and started my own fitness business called Personally Fit, Inc. The first facility was located in Rancho Santa Fe, an upscale coastal community near San Diego. My intent was to develop a training program that would focus on body sculpting and conditioning for high-level aspiring athletes, but I quickly found that most of the sculpting candidates were looking for a magic pill—and aspiring athletes had no money. The people coming in the door were looking for a solution to nagging middle-age injuries that kept them from playing their weekend sports. Most of these conditions—tennis elbow, rotator cuff strain, stiff neck, low-back pain, hip, knee and ankle problems—were a result of poor conditioning and overuse syndrome. These were conditions I could do something about. Most participants were individuals aged 50 to 75 who were self-employed, semi-retired entrepreneurs and venture capitalists who wanted to keep working and be able to play hard in their spare time. Sound familiar? My customers would come in with a specific purpose and realize that they were going to have to get fit to prevent the problem from happening again. Based on this philosophy, I successfully opened a second facility in another part of San Diego.

Even though I eventually sold both of my facilities, like Ken, I'm not retiring, I'm refiring! That involves not only continuing to work one-on-one with clients but also coaching high school kids and consulting within the health care industry. I want to keep working and playing hard for at least another 20 years. Sound familiar again? I am a strong-willed member of the Boomer generation and hope to inspire others by sharing my experience of working with Ken on his fitness journey.

During the first week of November 2010, I got a voicemail message on my phone from Ken. After listening to the message, I thought, *Is it February already?*—not because the leaves were falling in San Diego, but because I was getting a request from Ken to begin his exercise program. Ken and I had been down this road many times before. In years past, on or about Groundhog Day, I would get "that call" from Ken. I knew that if he was contacting me this early, he must have a newfound commitment to exercise.

I wondered where that commitment was coming from. Through the years I have found that there are three reasons or purposes that help people keep their commitment to their commitment to lead a healthy lifestyle.

The first is a *health-driven purpose*. I remember a cartoon I saw some time ago that shows a doctor talking to his overweight and unhealthy-looking patient. The doctor tells the patient, "Would you rather exercise for 1 hour a day or be dead for 24 hours a day?" Very funny, but you get the point. If the alternative to exercise is poor health or worse, you have a pretty powerful purpose.

The second is a *cause-driven purpose*—focusing on something greater than you. Last year my son Deyl decided he wanted to run the Sahara 150. This is an event where you run a marathon a day for four days, and then two marathons on the fifth day over the sand dunes of the Sahara Desert in 118-degree heat. Deyl had done triathlons and a marathon before, but never in such extreme conditions. Knowing he needed a purpose greater than just wanting to do it to say he'd completed it, he decided to make it a fund-raiser with the goal of raising $40,000 for the poor. He told me that without that great purpose, there were several times during the grueling race when he might have quit. He not only completed the race but exceeded his fund-raising goal.

The last, and most difficult, is a *personally driven purpose*. Why is it the most difficult? Because it often has a short-term goal attached to it and doesn't really involve much lifestyle change. An example would be the mother wanting to lose 30 pounds for her daughter's upcoming wedding so she looks good in the pictures. The weight loss is usually achieved, but the reversal begins at the wedding reception. The purpose for the weight loss is gone because old habits return, and the weight that's lost is usually gained back. Ken had experienced similar motivations in the past and frequently achieved short-term goals only to see them disappear. The main reason for this was that he always was doing it for the wrong purpose. I needed to know what was different this time.

When Ken and I got together in November, I asked him why he was so interested in starting a program at this time. He told me about his desire to avoid knee surgery, pressure from Scott, Margie, other members of his family, and colleagues who wanted him to focus on his health and fitness so he would be around much longer, and his own desire to see his grandkids grow up, mature, and graduate from college. He also told me about "the famous Joy." Realizing he couldn't do it by himself, Ken wanted to know what it would take to make me as committed to his success as he was. I told him that I could make the time, but it had to be for the right reasons—that his motivation to improve his fitness had to eventually come from within. In other words, *he must be doing this for himself, not for his loved ones.*

PRINCIPLE 2
Establish a Mutual Commitment to Success

As Ken already suggested, it is difficult for people to make a major change in their overall fitness routine by themselves. They need someone else—whether it be a family member, friend, colleague, or fitness coach like me—to help them keep their commitment to their commitment. How do you determine who that person should be? First, it should be someone who really cares about you and your individual success. Equally important, they have to be willing to hold you accountable, which sometimes requires tough love.

That means you not only have to *like* the person; you also have to *trust* them. Ken has always been one of my favorite people, and I really wanted him to be around for the long haul. Fortunately, he trusts me, which is very important, and enjoys my company. To top it off, we both agreed that keeping Ken committed to a program would be a challenge. With that thought in our minds, all we had to do was establish a mutual incentive.

After giving it considerable thought, I told Ken that what I wanted was the right to tell the story of his success—in simple words, that he and I would write a book together sharing all of the details.

As Ken thought about it, he realized that if he agreed to write a book with me, he would have my total commitment—because without success in our program, we would have no story to tell and there would be no book. With that, we shook hands and started to work.

Follow along with Ken and me as we begin this journey together. I think you'll enjoy the ride.

FOOD FOR THOUGHT

What is the health-driven, cause-driven, or personally driven purpose that motivates you toward a new goal?

Who is a person in your life whom you like and trust who could be as committed to your success as you are?

What kind of mutual incentive could you and this key person agree upon that would ensure your success?

The Launching Pad

Determining Appropriate Help: Learning About Situational Leadership® II

Ken: As I suggested in the introduction, at some time in our life we all have made a New Year's resolution to do something and then not followed through—we didn't behave on our good intentions. Most New Year's resolutions don't work because we find accomplishing the goal to be tougher than we thought it would be. Added to that, we get little, if any, help from people around us when we get discouraged. In fact, they often smile and say, "We'll believe it when we see it," and then walk away to let us manage on our own. But if we could do it by ourselves, it would not need to be a New Year's resolution—we would just do it.

PRINCIPLE 3
Learn About Situational Leadership® II

I knew right away that I could not regain my fitness on my own—a delegating leadership style wouldn't work

27

for me. Then I had a blinding flash of the obvious: Why not use Situational Leadership® II[1]—the model that has built our business more than anything else we have ever taught— to help Tim and me figure out the kind of leadership (i.e., help) I would need to accomplish the fitness goals we would agree upon?

That would be perfect because Situational Leadership® II—also known as SLII®—contends that leadership is not something you do *to* people; it's something you do *with* people. And if Tim and I both knew and practiced SLII®, he could give me the help I needed on each part of my fitness program. After all, according to SLII®, there is no one best leadership style for helping people to accomplish their goals. So a delegating style might work in some situations, but certainly not in an area where someone was struggling like I was with certain aspects of my fitness.

Three skills are necessary to effectively apply SLII® to any situation:

- Goal setting
- Diagnosing
- Matching

Goal Setting

All good performance starts with clear goals. After all, the first secret of *The One Minute Manager* is One Minute Goals. If

---

1. I first started developing Situational Leadership® in the late 1960s with Paul Hersey at Ohio University when we were writing our textbook *Management of Organizational Behavior*. In the 1980s when Margie and I began to build our own training and development business, together with our founding associates, we began to find that some critical aspects of Hersey's and my original Situational Leadership® model didn't fit the research on team development and observations about how most people feel when they are initially working on a new task or job. It was at that point we created Situational Leadership® II. See *Leadership and the One Minute Manager* (New York: HarperCollins, 1985 and 2013).

you don't know what you want to accomplish, there is very little chance you will get there.

In setting clear goals, it is important that the goals you set are SMART goals. SMART is an acronym to help you remember the key aspects of an effective goal. However, you should write your actual goals in this order: S, then T, then R, A, and M. I'll explain as we continue.

> **S** *stands for specific.* Goals should state exactly what you want to accomplish and when you want to accomplish it.
>
> **T** *stands for trackable.* How are you going to measure your performance? In other words, what are the performance standards? What does a good job look like?

So you first decide exactly what you want to achieve—S—and then you determine how you are going to track or measure progress toward goal accomplishment—T. Once the S and T are in place, then use the other three SMART criteria—the R, A, and M—to check if the goal is truly SMART.

> **R** *stands for relevant.* Is it really important? Will it make a difference in your life?
>
> **A** *stands for attainable.* Goals have to be reasonable. Whether or not they are reasonable depends on what has happened in the past. You want to stretch yourself but don't want to make a goal so difficult that it's unattainable and you lose commitment.
>
> **M** *stands for motivating.* For you to do your best work, the goals that are set need to tap into what you enjoy doing or know you will eventually enjoy doing.

Diagnosing

Once SMART goals are set—aligning what needs to be done and when—the next skill for using SLII® is diagnosing your development level on a specific goal or task.

Development level is a function of competence (skills/ experience) and commitment (motivation/confidence). In other words, any time you are not performing well, it is usually a competence problem, a commitment problem, or both.

Competence is a function of demonstrated knowledge and skills, which can be gained through learning or experience. When it came to fitness, I knew a lot about it—at least some aspects of it—having written about it and having been a part of a number of health and fitness programs. I have always had less of a competence problem than a commitment problem.

Commitment is a combination of confidence and motivation. Confidence is a measure of your self-assuredness—the feeling of being able to do a task with little help. Over the years, my confidence level to maintain a fitness program had eroded.

Motivation is a measure of your interest in and enthusiasm for doing a task well. There are times when you have the competence and confidence to do something, but no interest. Over the years, I lost motivation when I realized that living a healthy, fit lifestyle was going to be harder than I thought. I also found that I got bored with exercising and eating the right food. Some people lose motivation because they feel their efforts and progress aren't being acknowledged—in other words, they need other people's support and cheerleading. That certainly was true for me—and the reason why a delegating, leave-alone leadership style never worked for me in this area.

As you can imagine, there are different combinations of competence and commitment. To be precise, four combinations of competence and commitment make up what we call the four development levels. See the figure at the top of the next page.

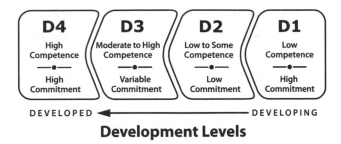

Development Levels

When you are a D1 on a particular goal or task, you are what we call an *enthusiastic beginner*. Even though you have high commitment, you are inexperienced because you are new to the task or goal. In many ways, *you don't know what you don't know*. Therefore, you are low on competence.

If you ever started a fitness program in the beginning of the year, I would imagine you were an enthusiastic beginner unless you had been down this road before, like me. Then you might be a D2, or what we call a *disillusioned learner*. You have low to some competence, because you have some prior knowledge and experience in the area you're working on. But you are discouraged because you haven't made as much progress as you expected. It's at this stage you could become frustrated and might even be ready to quit. That's what happened to me in my past fitness journeys. It happens to a lot of people.

If you are a D3, you are what we call a *capable but cautious performer*. You have demonstrated some competence and experience in doing the task, but lack confidence in doing that task by yourself. In that case, you can become self-critical and unsure. You can also become bored with a particular goal or task at this stage and lose commitment that way.

You ultimately hope to become a D4 in doing a task, and then you'll be what we call a *self-reliant achiever.* You will have both high competence and commitment and not require a New Year's resolution to perform well.

Besides knowing about the four different development levels, it is important to realize that *development is task- or goal-specific.* Since goal setting focuses your energy, make sure you don't set too many goals and dilute your efforts.

Once you have agreed upon three to five SMART goals in a particular area such as fitness, it is important that you analyze your development level on each of the agreed-upon goals. For example, you might be an avid jogger, and when it comes to aerobic exercise you are a D4—self-reliant achiever. But when it comes to nutrition and weight control, you are a D2—disillusioned learner. You are frustrated because you are constantly fighting your weight.

As a result, it was important for me—and it might be important for you—to realize that with a fitness program, you need different leadership styles, or help, for different parts of your program. If you are in good shape when it comes to aerobic exercise, you can be left alone and will continue to perform well, but if that same approach is used around nutrition and weight control, you will be in trouble.

Matching

This brings us to the third skill needed to use SLII®: Matching. This involves finding someone who can provide you with the appropriate amount of directive behavior and supportive behavior that you need to accomplish a goal.

- *Directive behavior* involves telling people what, when, where, and how to do things, and then closely observing them.

- *Supportive behavior* involves listening, praising, facilitating, interacting with, and involving people in decision making.

When I think about the difference between directive and supportive behavior, I go back to my days at the University of Massachusetts when I did a lot of work with teachers. We taught them that if a student came to a learning experience with their barrel *empty* of knowledge, the job of the teacher was to fill up that barrel. Directive behavior is a "barrel-filling" leadership style. If the student came to a learning experience with their barrel *full* of knowledge, the job of the teacher was to draw that knowledge out of the student and help them organize it in a way that made sense. Supportive behavior is a "barrel-drawing-out" leadership style.

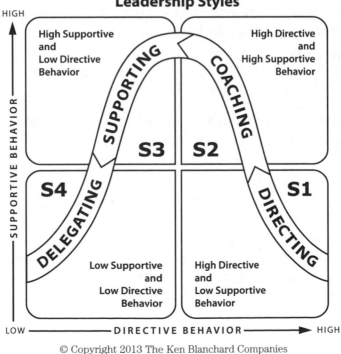

© Copyright 2013 The Ken Blanchard Companies

Just like with competence and commitment, there are four different combinations of directive and supportive behavior that make up the four leadership styles, as seen in the figure on the previous page:

Style 1—Directing: High Directive Behavior and Low Supportive Behavior
The leader provides specific direction about goals, shows and tells how, and closely tracks the individual's performance in order to provide frequent feedback on results.

Style 2—Coaching: High Directive Behavior and High Supportive Behavior
The leader continues to direct goal or task accomplishment but also explains why, solicits suggestions, and begins to encourage involvement in decision making.

Style 3—Supporting: Low Directive Behavior and High Supportive Behavior
The leader and the individual make decisions together. The role of the leader is to facilitate, listen, draw out, encourage, and support.

Style 4—Delegating: Low Directive Behavior and Low Supportive Behavior
The individual makes most of the decisions about what, how, and when. The role of the leader is to value the individual's contributions and support their growth.

How do these four leadership styles differ in terms of the "barrel-filling" and "barrel-drawing-out" concepts? Suppose when it comes to flexibility, you suddenly realize how important it is for your overall physical functioning. If a trainer or a knowledgeable friend were using an S1—Directing style with you on your flexibility, that person would tell you what your goal should be and what a good job would look like, and then closely supervise your performance. So S1—Directing is a "barrel-filling" style.

If someone were to use an S2—Coaching style with you on your flexibility, they would still be in charge and provide a lot of direction, but this is where a good trainer or knowledgeable friend would begin to engage in two-way communication by asking for your suggestions. This would involve providing a lot of support, because some of the ideas you suggest would be good—and it would be important for an S2 leader to reinforce your initiative and capacity to start to evaluate your own efforts. So an S2—Coaching leadership style is both a "barrel-filling" and "barrel-drawing-out" style.

If a trainer or knowledgeable friend wanted to use an S3—Supporting leadership style with you on your flexibility, that person would keep the ball in your court—supporting your efforts, listening to your suggestions, and asking questions to build your confidence in your competence. Rarely would an S3 leader talk about how to go about accomplishing a particular task. Such a leader would instead help you reach your own solution by asking questions to expand thinking and encourage risk taking. So an S3—Supporting leadership style is a "barrel-drawing-out" style.

If someone working with you on your flexibility wanted to use an S4—Delegating leadership style, that person would turn over to you the responsibility for day-to-day decision making and problem solving on building your flexibility. So with an S4—Delegating leadership style, there is little "barrel filling" *or* "barrel drawing out" taking place.

So you can see how, with the same task—improving your flexibility—a trainer or knowledgeable friend can use any of the four leadership styles.

Once you know what areas you need to work on—such as aerobic exercise, strength, flexibility, or balance training, or nutrition/weight control—you are ready to find someone like Tim who can match the appropriate leadership style to your development level in each area. In other words, to help you achieve a goal, a trainer or knowledgeable friend not only needs to use *different strokes for different folks,* but also *different strokes for the same folks on different goals.*

Take a look at our complete Situational Leadership® II model on the next page. To determine the appropriate leadership style you need, imagine a vertical line from your development level up into the style portion of the model. Where that line hits the curve running through the four leadership styles will indicate the appropriate leadership style required for your development level. So, as the illustration indicates:

S1—Directing is for *enthusiastic beginners* who lack competence but are enthusiastic and committed (D1). They need direction and frequent feedback to get them started and to develop their competence.

S2—Coaching is for *disillusioned learners* who have some competence but lack commitment (D2). They need direction and feedback because they're still relatively inexperienced. They also need support and acknowledgement to build their self-confidence and motivation, and involvement in decision making to restore their commitment.

S3—Supporting is for *capable but cautious performers* who have competence but lack confidence or

Situational Leadership® II Model

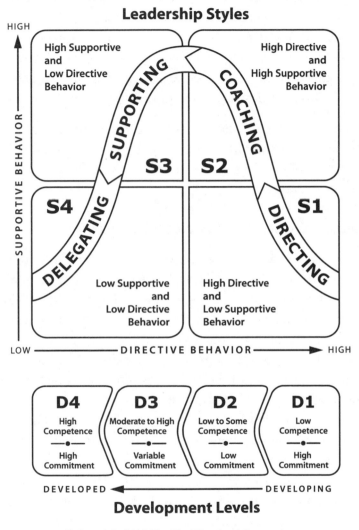

Leadership Styles

Development Levels

motivation (D3). They do not need much direction because of their skills, but support is necessary to bolster their confidence and motivation.

S4—Delegating is for *self-reliant achievers* who have both competence and commitment (D4). They are able and willing to work on a project by themselves with little direction or support.

Because we will be referring to the concepts in Situational Leadership® II throughout the rest of the book, we have reproduced this model on the last page of the book for your easy reference.

Changing Leadership Style over Time

Once you and a trainer or knowledgeable friend have determined which leadership style to use on each area of your fitness program, the question becomes this: Does the trainer always use the same style on a particular area? The answer is no. The goal is to move your development level to the point where an S4—Delegating leadership style would work. In my case, I would then be competent and committed to effectively carry on without Tim's supervision. As you'll see throughout our journey, Tim doesn't do just a one-time diagnosis of my development level and deliver the appropriate style. He is always looking for opportunities to move forward on the leadership style curve from S1—Directing, where I was an enthusiastic beginner, to S2—Coaching, if any disillusionment set in, and then to S3—Supporting, where I needed more support than direction, and eventually—ideally—to S4—Delegating, where I was able to manage my own performance. In a sense, you have to look at the curve running through the model as a railroad track. If you start at station

S1—Directing and you want to get to S4—Delegating, you have to stop at S2—Coaching and S3—Supporting before you get there.

Problems occur when you skip a style. The most serious error you can make is to have someone start off directing your effort (S1) and then, for some reason, that person stops working with you and leaves you alone (S4) to work on accomplishing a goal by yourself. In many ways, I made that mistake in the past when I got too busy with travel and forced Tim to jump off the track and go directly to an inappropriate S4—Delegating leadership style. If you look at the model, you'll notice there is no railroad track that goes straight from S1—Directing to S4—Delegating. What happens if a train goes off the track? People get hurt—they get discouraged and don't accomplish their goals.

To illustrate the importance of staying on the leadership railroad track when helping someone accomplish a goal or goals, let me relate my experience teaching golf.

Just a minute, Blanchard, we already heard about your basketball coaching. What is this about teaching golf?

My favorite sport besides basketball is golf. My dad introduced me to the game at about the same time he put a basket in our basement—when I was six years old. I never met a golf game I didn't like.

In 1984, I got a call from Jerry Tarde, editor of *Golf Digest* magazine. He had just finished reading *The One Minute Manager* and was intrigued by the analogy we drew in the book suggesting that not providing clear goals for people was like asking them to play golf at night—in both cases, they wouldn't perform very well because they wouldn't be able to see the pins (i.e., goals).

Jerry asked me if I played golf.

I was quick to reply, "I'm a golf nut."

He was delighted and asked if I would write an article with one of their top teaching pros entitled *The One Minute Golfer*.

I said I would be happy to do the article if I could coauthor it with a pro named Bob Toski, because I had heard he was a great golf teacher and also quite a character. So I flew to Florida and spent two days writing with Bob. Our article appeared as the cover story in the June 1985 issue of *Golf Digest* magazine. It went over so well that Jerry asked me to go to one of their golf schools and write a follow-up article entitled *The One Minute Manager Goes to Golf School*. As a result, I spent a fun week in Alabama working and playing with Toski and other esteemed golf teachers.

I didn't end up writing the article, however. Why? Because I learned that at most golf schools the instructors use mainly S1—Directing and S2—Coaching leadership styles throughout the program. Then, when school is over, they go straight to an S4—Delegating style. As a result, the students often get worse after they leave because they have "paralysis by analysis" and can't put what they learned into practice on their own. So I decided to co-found The Golf University® in the San Diego area with some local golf pros.

At the beginning of our two-and-a-half day school, I would teach all of the students SLII® so they could understand the journey we would be taking them on. The first morning, our pros would analyze each student's golf game and set three or four learning goals for their time with us. Then the pros used S1—Directing and S2—Coaching styles with their students for the rest of the day. Rather than rotating everyone around the same learning stations in an attempt to teach them everything about golf in one school, we divided the students into groups with similar goals based on their golf experience.

The second day, our pros predominantly used S2—Coaching and S3—Supporting styles with the students on their learning goals. On the final morning, when students hit a shot, their pros would not comment about the shot until the students had analyzed their own performance. Why? Because the pros knew that when the school ended, the students would be forced to go to an S4—Delegating leadership style. Unless the students could direct and support themselves on what they had learned, they would not improve and might even get worse after graduation. Having our pros stay on the leadership railroad track—moving from S1, to S2, to S3 during school, to the inevitable S4 style at the end of the program—worked well as students continued to improve.

Quite a few retirees, who had never played before but wanted to learn the game, came to our school once each quarter for a year or so. Each time they came, we would give them new learning goals, work them through the railroad track again with these new goals from S1, to S2, to S3, and then send them home with the S4—Delegating style and they would practice what they had learned. After several visits to the school, a number of these "beginner seniors" ended up shooting in the low 80s or high 70s. With results like that, we were named one of the top golf schools in America under the leadership of our head pro, Tom Wischmeyer.

We closed The Golf University® after 9/11 when people just weren't traveling anymore to noncritical activities like golf schools. But using SLII® and changing our leadership style over time as a strategy for improving students' golf games really worked. In fact, I wrote a book about the process, originally entitled *Playing the Great Game of Golf: Making Every Minute Count* and later retitled *The One Minute Golfer: Enjoy the Great Game More*.

Why have I taken so much time in this section to talk about Situational Leadership® II? Because SLII® concepts are vital to understanding how to move forward and accomplish goals—whether it be with your golf game or anything else—as I was attempting to do with my fitness program. The reason I had failed so often in the past was that I hadn't allowed either myself or Tim to practice what I preached. I had cut off Tim's support and direction too early when I obviously couldn't handle an S4—Delegating leadership style yet.

With my newfound awareness that SLII® would have a big part in my fitness journey, it was time for me to commit to my commitment. As you go on this journey with Tim and me, you will see that the concepts from Situational Leadership® II come into play continually.

FOOD FOR THOUGHT

Create your own SLII® story: To illustrate how you have probably utilized the concepts in Situational Leadership® II throughout your life even without knowing it, think of a time when you had a goal to learn something that you are now great at doing (D4) but at one time you could not do at all. Examples would be riding a bicycle, learning a new language, or kicking a bad habit. Describe what you felt and what you did at each stage of development:

(Continued next page)

D1—enthusiastic beginner: Before you actually started the activity or behavior—you were thinking about doing it, were getting ready to start, or you had just begun to work on it

D2—disillusioned learner: When you really wanted to quit doing the activity or behavior, or were frustrated

D3—capable but cautious performer: When you could do the activity or behavior, but weren't consistently confident about your ability to do it

D4—self-reliant achiever: When the task was easy and you could do it without any supervision; you could mentor others

Establishing Areas of Focus: Preparing for the Yearlong Program

Tim: Even though Ken and I had worked together many times in the past, this was the first time I had committed to total hands-on involvement, being just as responsible for the short- and long-term results as Ken. Given that, we both agreed that November—before we officially started the formal one-year program—should be directed toward establishing the fitness areas we would focus on and determining the appropriate help Ken would need from me in each area to accomplish our agreed-upon goals.

PRINCIPLE 4
Develop Age-Appropriate Goals

My first concern was what kind of exercise Ken should be doing at his age. I have been in the fitness industry for over 40 years and have noticed that many physiological changes occur through a normal lifetime.

My first realization of the inevitability of age-related physiological differences occurred when I was 45. A track enthusiast friend of mine convinced me that I should compete in masters-level track and field competitions. Since I was in great shape and very strong for my age, I decided to compete in the shot put. I threw well in college, and when I saw that the All American standard was only 41 feet, I got very excited. I threw so hard trying to reach that mark that I pulled a hamstring muscle. I couldn't believe that I was throwing nearly 20 feet less than I threw when I was in college. I knew age brought certain physiological changes, but how could it make such a difference?

As we get older, our bones become more brittle, our joint cartilages wear thinner, and our ligaments become looser. Sounds kind of depressing, doesn't it? The good news is that we have the same muscle cells regenerating and will for as long as we use them. What this means from a training standpoint is that we can't handle the exercise demands that we once did.

The objective of my first month working with Ken was to initially provide him with a basic orientation on the six components of a complete, age-appropriate fitness program. Then, using Situational Leadership® II, we would determine the appropriate leadership style I needed to use on each component to help him succeed.

Why all this planning? Because, unfortunately, most people have a philosophy of "ready-fire-aim" rather than "ready-aim-fire." They want to get started before they know where they're going and how they're going to get there.

Let's take a look at the six components of a complete fitness program.

Aerobic Exercise

Aerobic exercise occurs when oxygen combines with fat and carbohydrate to form ATP (adenosine triphosphate) for muscle fuel. Aerobic exercise has numerous benefits: The heart muscle gets stronger, lung capacity improves, mitochondria (muscle cells) increase in number, circulation improves, and we can burn stored body fat. Other major benefits of a good aerobic program are increased capillaries, greater energy level, and stress relief. A number of studies show that aerobic exercise is good for the brain—particularly cognitive function and memory retention. Some studies have even indicated that it may delay the onset of Alzheimer's disease. All of these benefits will make us healthier—and aerobic exercise is relatively simple to do.

I am very familiar with Ken's capabilities and limitations because I have worked with him for so many years. When it comes to aerobic exercise, we both diagnosed him as a D2—disillusioned learner. He had some success in the past through basketball and also with jogging when he first came to California, but he was frustrated that he could not maintain a consistent aerobic routine. Given that diagnosis, I had to set up a program that was challenging yet realistic for Ken—and not boring. In coaching him in this area, I needed to take the lead in setting up his program but also seek his suggestions and involvement; an S2—Coaching leadership style.

Ken had completed his rehab from a second total hip replacement six months earlier. He had been doing about 15 minutes of aerobic exercise on his recumbent bike at home two to three times per week. This was very minimal, but at least he was getting some exercise stimulus. I knew that his aerobic exercise would be limited to cycling because of a limitation with his left knee. A basketball injury (Ken claims he hit his knee on the rim) and a subsequent knee surgery in 1961 had resulted in a knee condition that was very arthritic and lacked full extension by at least 15 degrees. This left Ken with the equivalent of a shorter left leg and was partially responsible for the "Quasimodo" look that his son Scott was concerned about. Walking any distance was not directly painful but caused other problems with spinal displacement and posture.

My objective for the first month was to have him work out on his exercise bike a minimum of 15 minutes at 100 to 115 heartbeats per minute (bpm), twice a day for at least five days per week. The goal would be to eventually combine those two 15-minute sessions into one 30-minute session at that same heart rate once a day. Ken could continue to do this at home on his own, with me monitoring him closely and cheering his progress.

Strength Training

Strength training has always been my favorite component of fitness. Muscle tissue is one of the only body tissues that continues to regenerate over a lifetime. However, you are only as strong as you need to be to do your daily activities.

When muscle tissue grows, the term is *hypertrophy*. When muscle tissue shrinks, it is called *atrophy*. Both conditions can occur rather quickly. If you have ever had a limb in a cast for six weeks, you've probably observed how quickly tissues shrink when they are immobilized. When people retire, they often spend too much time sitting around and rapidly lose the strength of their stabilizer muscles. This is why many older adults have trouble with balance. Some people worry that strength training will develop large bulky muscles. The reality is that they should worry more about losing too much muscle. Numerous studies have cited that adults who don't engage in strength training will lose an average of one-half pound of lean muscle tissue per year after age 25.

In terms of strength training, Ken was a D1—enthusiastic beginner. He never really had done any strength training but was excited about becoming a little buff—at least enough to get a "You're looking good" from Margie. Given his lack of experience in strength training along with his enthusiasm to give it a try, I needed to provide an S1—Directing leadership style. My job was to design a program for Ken and closely supervise him to avoid any potential injury. His job was to do what I said.

Ken started to come to my facility two to three times per week to do strength training. Initially, we worked for about 45 minutes each session. I divided his strength training program into upper-body, lower-body, and trunk exercises. Most of the upper-body exercises were done initially on a cable-driven multi-gym machine from a sitting position. It was easier for him to do these exercises as they did not require a lot of body stabilizing and balance. Also, the cables operate independently, which allows the limbs to work together to correct any bilateral deficiency. Ken's legs were exercised on a Pilates Reformer, and his trunk was exercised on a massage table. I placed a lot of emphasis on proper form, correct breathing, and doing the full range of motion. The goal for each exercise was to achieve muscular fatigue at 15 reps for upper body, 20 to 25 reps for the leg muscles, and as many as 40 reps for the torso exercises.

Flexibility

This is my least favorite component of the exercise regime. However, it is as important as the others. A flexibility program can be completed in 10 to 15 minutes and ideally should be done daily or at least every time after you work out. As we get older and spend less time actively moving around, the muscles become tighter and shorter, thus restricting our ability to move around and increasing the chance of injury.

In terms of flexibility, Ken was a D2—disillusioned learner. Periodically he would go to his local Egoscue clinic and see Pete Egoscue or one of his staff. Pete was a Vietnam veteran who had trouble standing up straight after returning from his tour of duty. So he decided to learn about the body, resulting in the Egoscue Method®, which specializes in alignment. But like Weight Watchers, Ken would start a program with the Egoscue folks with great enthusiasm and then get too busy to follow through. As a result, I decided to do flexibility work with Ken along with his strength training at my facility, where I could direct his efforts and encourage his progress: an S2—Coaching leadership style.

It became clear to me that flexibility was an area where Ken would need a lot of work. Years of poor postural alignment, mostly related to his knee condition, had resulted in him having very tight muscles. Most of the strength training exercises were done with as much range of motion as possible to help free up the movement of the joints. Strength training work was done first, since warm muscles move better than cold muscles. The majority of the stretching exercises were done by me manually moving his limbs. One of the objectives was to make Ken capable of eventually doing his own stretching.

Balance Training

Balance begins to decline in your late 20s and gets progressively worse from age 60 on. For most people, this is of little consequence until the later years, when it can result in falls as well as hip and arm fractures. A lot of this balance deficiency is the result of weaker stabilizer muscles from less activity, and some is due to loss of proprioception.

Proprioception is the body's ability to compensate for gravity and that third plane of movement. It is a coordinated effort among the brain, muscles, and joints to react to movement that might cause us to fall. A simple example is what occurs when we walk or step off a curb. We do not consciously have to think about where we need to place our foot to maintain balance, as our body does that automatically.

Another system that affects our balance is the vestibular system. This mostly involves the fluid in our inner ear and is largely responsible for maintaining our equilibrium. A number of things can cause problems with the vestibular system, and most require medical intervention. The other two balance factors mentioned—weak stabilizer muscles and gradual loss of proprioception—can be improved by training.

When it came to balance training, again Ken was a D1—enthusiastic beginner. He hadn't thought much about the importance of balance but was quick to get excited about it when I convinced him of the consequences of lack of balance when we age. Using an S1—Directing leadership style, I had Ken attempt to balance himself standing on one foot while he was looking straight ahead—first his left foot and then his right. I also had him stand on a BOSU® ball—a quarter-round ball with a flat bottom—with me not holding on, but close enough to catch him when he lost his balance. Showing improvement with these activities I knew would go a long way in building up Ken's balance.

Nutrition and Weight Control

We've all heard the expression "You are what you eat." If you mainly eat fat, you are generally fat. If you eat starches and simple sugars—much of which are converted to fat—you are usually fat. If you eat what your body requires with the correct amounts and types of proteins, carbohydrates, and fats, you can become a "lean, mean (not necessarily) fighting machine."

When it comes to nutrition and weight control, I'm sure by now you could diagnose Ken's development level yourself. Given his yo-yo history and in-and-out forays with the Weight Watchers program, he was definitely a D2—disillusioned learner.

Ken and I discussed several weight loss options. His first thought was to rejoin Weight Watchers, where he had achieved some success in the past. While I wanted to support him here, I did remind him of how often he had gained weight back after he stopped attending the meetings. As a result, I directed him first to consult with Sabrina Zaslov, the nutrition advisor in Dr. Rice's office, on an eating and nutrition program. After that, the Weight Watchers program and the cheering of the fellow participants at the meetings could complement and support any progress made and hopefully provide the S2—Coaching leadership style he needed.

Rest and Sleep

Most adults are sleep deprived, causing marked reduction in their productivity, concentration, and quality of work. Several leading Fortune 500 companies and professional associations, as well as professional sports teams, are learning that it is neither macho nor smart to operate on less than the required amount of sleep.

This was one area where Ken didn't really need any help. In fact, he told me that Dr. James B. Maas, an expert on sleep and performance and a personal friend of Ken's since graduate school, had made an appointment for him at the sleep clinic at UCSD Medical School to do a routine test, which Ken passed with flying colors. According to the attending physician, Ken broke the record as the person who fell asleep most quickly! Ken was certainly a D4—self-reliant achiever in terms of rest and sleep. This was one part of his health and fitness program where an S4—Delegating leadership style worked just fine.

FOOD FOR THOUGHT

Do you have a story about a time when you realized you couldn't do a physical task as well as you could when you were 18 or 20?

Where are you in terms of development level (D1, D2, D3, or D4) on the six components of your own fitness program:

- Aerobic exercise?
- Strength training?
- Flexibility?
- Balance training?
- Nutrition and weight control?
- Rest and sleep?

Which area or areas do you feel need the most work?

What would you have to give up to get one more hour of sleep every night? Think about whether it would be worth that sacrifice to be able to function at a higher level and have more energy every day.

Setting Goals to Monitor Progress

Ken: Once Tim and I had agreed on the six areas everyone should focus on in a fitness program, and determined my development level in each area and the appropriate leadership style (help) I would need, it made sense for us to initiate an evaluation process. Why? Because goal accomplishment involves moving from an *actual* level of performance to a *desired* level of performance. Your actual level of performance at the beginning of any program is referred to as *baseline data.*

An important truth I've learned over the years is if you can't measure something, you can't manage it. Gathering observable, measurable baseline data from Tim in the fitness area and from Dr. Rice in the medical/physical area would not only permit us to set goals—the first secret of *The One Minute Manager*—but also allow us to monitor progress. Monitoring progress is key. Once goals were set, we would be able to observe my measurable results so that initially Tim could praise my progress and, if appropriate, change the leadership style he was using on a particular area. Eventually the goal would be for me to praise my own progress. After all, the second secret of *The One Minute Manager* is One Minute Praisings.

Monitoring progress would also allow Tim to redirect my efforts when progress was not being made. The third secret of *The One Minute Manager* is One Minute Reprimands, which today we prefer to call One Minute Redirects. When redirection is appropriate, it might signal a need to move backward through the Situational Leadership® II curve from an S3—Supporting to an S2—Coaching leadership style.

On only a rare occasion—possibly when an injury occurs— would there be a need to move from an S4—Delegating style where the person had been a D4—self-reliant achiever back to an S3—Supporting style because the person was once again a D3—capable but cautious performer. At the same time, seldom would you find a D2—disillusioned learner reverting back to a D1—enthusiastic beginner requiring a movement from an S2—Coaching style back to an S1— Directing style. The only example I can think of for this would be if someone were completely frustrated with their progress and wanted to start over again at square one.

The reason all this is important for Tim's and my situation is that there are three aspects of managing performance:

1. *Performance planning*—where clear, observable, SMART goals are set, development level is diagnosed on each goal, and then the initial match of appropriate leadership style to use with each goal is determined.
2. *Day-to-day coaching*—where Situational Leadership® II is put into action by observing performance and delivering either praise or redirection, as well as potentially changing the leadership style being given.
3. *Performance evaluation*—where it is determined whether or not success was achieved. In other words, was each goal accomplished?

The step that is usually given the least focus is the second one—day-to-day coaching. People set goals and then work to accomplish them, but without day-to-day coaching, unless a person is a D4—self-reliant achiever on a goal or task, goal accomplishment will not be possible.

Fortunately, day-to-day coaching through an understanding of Situational Leadership® II, with Tim as my coach, was central to both of us accomplishing our goals—Tim's of being able to write a book about our successful fitness journey and mine of becoming fit again.

FOOD FOR THOUGHT

When was the last time you had a comprehensive fitness evaluation?

How can baseline data about your health and fitness help you set goals and monitor progress?

Why do you think day-to-day coaching is such an important aspect of managing performance?

Ken's Health and Fitness Evaluation

Tim: Prior to the first quarter's exercise program, which we started in December, I put Ken through an evaluation process. The first step was to review his health history. The most important purpose of the health history is to find out what, if any, medical conditions exist that would limit an exercise program. Since I had worked with Ken for so many years, the only thing I needed to do was to update his health history from the previous year. If he were a new client, I would have reviewed his complete health history to determine whether he needed to have a medical exam before proceeding.

The major changes in Ken's health history involved a total replacement of his second hip, which had been done the previous June, and a heart arrhythmia condition. I was very familiar with post–hip replacement limitations but felt that I should call Lee Rice, Ken's doctor, to see whether there were any limitations concerning his heart condition. Dr. Rice told me the arrhythmia situation had been resolved with a successful ablation treatment. (Note: *ablation* is a technique that essentially "disconnects" the source of the abnormal rhythm from the rest of the heart.)

Fitness Evaluation

I have always adjusted the format of my fitness evaluations to the individual being tested. As Ken mentioned, to monitor progress as the program moves along, it is always a good idea to take objective measurements at the outset. These measurements should be used to compare the fitness level of the individual to their own age group and, again, to establish a baseline on which progress can be measured. The following measurements are ones that I consider important and appropriate.

Body weight. I am not a big believer in stepping on the scale every week, because it is not a good measure of losing the right kind of weight. A good example occurred when I was a young captain at West Point being considered for promotion to major. I received a letter from the promotion board stating that while my service record was exemplary, I was overweight by army standards and might not be promoted unless I lost weight. I was 73 inches tall and weighed 210 pounds. By military standards, my weight should not have exceeded 188. According to those standards, I was

22 pounds overweight. Colonel James Anderson, the head of the physical education department, felt that it was time to get the military to change its standards, and I became the test case. He pointed out that while weighing 210 pounds, I had only 6 percent body fat, would ace every fitness test, and was the example of what a soldier should look like in uniform. The other side of his argument was that many soldiers within the weight standard were poor physical performers with very low muscle content. This experience led to a change of standards—the military would now consider body composition by also measuring the amount of body fat. To my delight, I ultimately was promoted. I believe that the weight scale should be used along with body fat measurement to serve as a marker as well as to determine body composition.

Ken's initial weight: 232 pounds (a bit pudgy). Goal: Below 200

Height. This measurement has many uses. We frequently hear people say, "I'm too short for my weight," or "I don't need to lose weight—I need to get taller." Whatever the case, we do accept that as we get older our height diminishes. Every year when I do my annual physical, I tell the nurse, "You're pressing the measuring planer too close to the top of my head"—a poor excuse for the fact that I am getting shorter. The reasons we actually get shorter have to do with joint cartilage wearing thinner, bone loss, and poor posture. While we can't yet replace cartilage, and we can't easily replace bone loss, we can definitely improve posture and stand taller and straighter.

Ken's initial height: 5'8" (Ken says he used to be 5'11". Some of that loss is postural.) Goal: 5'9".

Head distance from wall. This is where I have the individual stand back to the wall and chin level to the ground and measure the distance from the head to the wall. Many people begin to get a "hunched-over" look as they age, and this is the way to measure the severity of this problem. Sometimes it is occupationally driven. I've worked with a lot of dentists, surgeons, and computer operators who have spent years with their heads leaning forward and have subsequent neck problems. Most of these conditions are correctable with proper exercise.

Ken's initial measurement: 3.5" from the wall.
Goal: 2" from the wall.

Neck circumference. Fat accumulates here, sometimes forming a "second chin."

Ken's initial measurement: 17.0 inches.
Goal: 16-inch shirt rather than 17-inch.

Chest circumference, relaxed. Measured with a tape measure at nipple level.

Ken's initial measurement: 41.5 inches.
Goal: 40.5 inches.

Chest circumference, expanded. Measured in the same manner as above but with the individual inhaling and inflating the lungs with as much air as possible.

Ken's initial measurement: 42 inches. Goal: 41 inches.

Waist. Tape measurement at navel level.

Ken's initial measurement: 45 inches.
Goal: 40 inches. ("Get rid of 'fat pants.'")

Hips. Tape measurement at the largest point around the hips.

Ken's initial measurement: 46 inches.
Goal: 42 inches.

Upper arm/bicep, relaxed. Maximum girth measurement at midpoint of upper arm.

Ken's initial measurement: 14 inches.
Goal: 13 inches. ("Smaller guns.")

Upper arm/bicep, flexed. Maximum girth measurement at midpoint of upper arm.

Ken's initial measurement: 14 inches.
Goal: 14 inches. ("Firmer guns.")

Both thighs. Measured 7 inches above the knee.

Ken's initial measurement:

Right: 26 inches. Goal: 25 inches.

Left (arthritic knee): 24 inches. Goal: Less pain and 25 inches.

Hamstring flex. Measured with goniometer.

Right: Minus 35 degrees. Goal: Minus 15 degrees.

Left: Minus 45 degrees. Goal: Minus 30 degrees.

Goal: "Ability to do the limbo with younger people."

Heel cord. Measured with goniometer.

Right: 0 degrees. Goal: Minus 10 degrees.

Left: Minus 5 degrees. Goal: Minus 10 degrees.

Goal: "Ability to tap dance."—a definite D1 area for Ken!

Basic balance. Stand on one foot at a time; measured in seconds until balance is lost.

Right foot: 2 seconds. Goal: 30 seconds.

Left foot: 10 seconds. Goal: 30 seconds.

BOSU ball: 0 seconds.

Goal: To stand for 60 seconds "and swing a golf club."

Medical Exam

A medical exam is essential before starting an exercise program. Because exercise places a demand on the body, it is always a good idea to ensure that all systems are functioning normally. If not, you need to know what the limitations are. Dr. Rice has been Ken's primary care physician for the past 25 years and knows Ken's complete medical history. He conducts a physical exam at least once a year for each of his patients. Ken's annual exam was due, so the timing for this startup program was just right.

Dr. Rice's facility, the Lifewellness Institute in San Diego, conducts a very thorough exam that includes but is not limited to the following: family history, personal history, health habits, reviews of all systems, physical exam findings, significant test results, body fat percentage, cardiovascular testing, resting metabolic rate, ultrasound exam of major areas, bone density, pulmonary function, blood pressure, body weight, blood lipid profile, upper-body strength, abdominal strength, flexibility, and diet/nutrition.

The areas we feel are most relevant to Ken's fitness improvement, and his initial scores, are as follows:

Blood pressure: 116/72
Total cholesterol: 153
LDL cholesterol: 86
HDL cholesterol: 46
Cholesterol/HDL ratio: 3.3
Triglycerides: 107
Resting heart rate: 72
Sit-ups: 50 (2 minutes)
Push-ups: 9

Almost all of these areas are affected by a fitness program. Ken's physical exam included every aspect of health and fitness. In addition to what I tested, he had a nutritional analysis with a dietitian and a cardiovascular conditioning assessment by an exercise physiologist.

Although this type of exam is ideal, it can also be expensive—but some find that it is covered by their health insurance. At a minimum, you should visit your doctor and state that you intend to start a vigorous exercise program so that all necessary health areas can be checked.

Exercise coaches and personal trainers can be expensive as well; however, they are a good idea, at least to help you get started in the right direction and periodically check your progress. If your budget is an issue, many gyms and YMCAs offer occasional trainers for modest fees. How much is your health and fitness worth to you? Avoiding injury and sickness is economical in the long run.

Dr. Rice knew that I had worked with Ken for many years as his fitness coach, and he was very happy to learn that Ken and I were making a serious commitment to Ken's

fitness program. After the exam he made the following suggestions to Ken, which Ken shared with me:

- Work on a progressive aerobic program as established
  by Tim. Program intensity should be at a heart rate
  of 100 to 110 bpm. Include some interval training in
  your aerobic workout.
- Continue your weight training routine two to three
  times per week.
- Be sure to do some stretching every day.
- Continue your weight loss pursuit through the Weight
  Watchers program with advice from nutrition advisor Sabrina Zaslov along with a balanced and regular
  exercise program.

FOOD FOR THOUGHT

Not working with a fitness professional? Most of
the measurements Tim used in Ken's evaluation
can be done with a simple cloth measuring tape.
Before you begin your fitness journey, work with
a partner to document as many of these baseline
measurements as you can. Go ahead and take a
"before" photo for extra motivation and to monitor
progress!

If losing weight is one of your fitness goals, get
your doctor's opinion on the most appropriate and
sensible way for you to approach this part of your
program.

Selecting the Right Program for You

Tim: At this point you've heard all about Ken's program. What about you? We assume that if you have read this far, you are interested in how our journey might apply to you.

Several very important elements must be put in place when preparing for your own program.

Have a compelling purpose. Remember, whether you have a health-driven purpose, a cause-driven purpose, or a personally driven purpose, it must be *your purpose, not someone else's. You are doing this for yourself.*

Get a medical checkup. The American College of Sports Medicine suggests that any individual over age 40 should check with their physician prior to starting a vigorous exercise program. I would add that a sedentary individual of any age should do the same. This can range from a "minute clinic" visit to a full-fledged medical and physical exam such as Ken had at the Lifewellness Institute. The purpose for the medical checkup is to ensure that you don't have a medical condition that would prohibit or limit your participation.

Get educated about fitness. This is important because you need to understand what you are doing and why you are doing it. Fitness advice comes at us from everywhere in every form of media—books, magazines, TV programs, DVDs, the Internet, seminars, etc. Even my local newspaper has an entire section dedicated to fitness every Tuesday. Because a license is not required to teach or write about fitness, virtually everyone could call themselves professionals.

Be sure to do your homework before laying out your money or following someone's advice based on appearances or marketing hype. A consultation with a legitimate fitness professional can help guide you to the most appropriate information sources for your age and fitness level.

Establish goals. As with any other worthwhile project, it is necessary to set goals throughout your fitness program to achieve good results. Be sure your goals are SMART goals: Specific, Motivating, Attainable, Relevant, and Trackable. This is the time to pay a fitness professional for what they know. At a minimum, the person should have a bachelor's degree in sports science and experience in working with people of your age group.

For years, I offered people at this early stage a three-session startup. Each session was an hour in length. During the first session I would evaluate health history, do a simple fitness evaluation, discuss goals, and talk about the plan. In the second session I would present my recommendations and we would implement the plan. The third session was a one-month follow-up to see how the client was progressing. A startup plan such as this is an effective way to be sure you are beginning a program suitable for your specific needs and goals.

Set up a support system. Anytime you measure long-term success, the results are often only as good as your support system. An effective support system usually starts with a spouse or significant other, and the best scenario is when you are working on your fitness together. When this is not the case, at a minimum you need to have this person's genuine support—nothing is worse than when you are trying to eat a low-calorie, healthy meal and your spouse or closest friend is sitting across from you eating a cheeseburger and fries!

If you don't have a significant other who is part of your fitness program, try to identify another reliable workout partner. Ideally, this should be someone who has the same goals you have and—most important—someone who is at least as motivated as you are. I always find that when I play golf with golfers who are worse than me, I play poorly. When I play with golfers who are better than me, I play better. Choose wisely!

The rest of your support team can include family members, friends, and work colleagues who have your best interests at heart.

Use Situational Leadership® II to ensure success. When I started my fitness business in 1987 and opened my first facility, my goal was member retention. Because the Situational Leadership® II model in many ways is common-sense organized, even before I knew the formal concept, I used it when people would join my program. I believed it was important to put each member on the program at a level at which they were most likely to succeed. This approach was very effective—my clubs had a retention rate of better than 90 percent with no contracts.

Here are some examples of real people at different development levels and the kind of help (i.e., leadership style) they needed.

D1—Enthusiastic Beginner (Low Competence/High Commitment). A 45-year-old woman who was 50 pounds overweight joined my program. She said her doctor had told her she must lose weight or she could face serious health problems. She had tried dieting alone with little success and wanted to try exercise but hated it. I asked her what type of exercise she could tolerate, and she said that she enjoyed walking but for many reasons couldn't do it when she got home from work. She worked next door to our fitness facility and took an hour for lunch.

After assessing her, I found that she was willing to walk every day, and she loved to read. I explained how aerobic exercise alone could really help (details in the Resources II section), and she began her workouts the next day. Initially, under the watchful eye of one of our staff members, she would walk on the treadmill for 45 minutes each day while reading a book. Then she added an hour on the weekends. After three months she had lost 12 pounds, within six months she had lost 28 pounds and after a full year she was down 48 pounds. As time went on, she needed minimal S1—Directing or S2—Coaching, but she continued to get lots of S3—Supporting style from staff and other members. By year's end, she had progressed from D1 to D4 and was taking exercise classes and doing strength training. She and her doctor were both very happy.

D2—Disillusioned Learner (Low to Some Competence/ Low Commitment). A 50-year-old man who was recovering from a serious stroke joined the facility. The left side of his body was mostly paralyzed, and his medical coverage for stroke rehab had ended because he had stopped making progress. He could drive a car and was fully retired on disability.

He desperately needed exercise but could not afford a full-time trainer. After assessing him, I realized that he had been a D2—disillusioned learner for some time but now had a very distinct purpose. He could do the exercise bike on his own and do minimal strength training—but what he desperately needed was stretching, which he could not do by himself. I arranged to have him stretched twice per week for 30 minutes by a trainer. He is still dedicated to his program after 20 years. Even though he had only marginal improvement of the paralysis, his quality of life improved immensely. He comes for his workout five times per week on his own, and with staff help he has progressed from a D1/D2 to a D4.

D3—Capable but Cautious Performer (Moderate to High Competence/Variable Commitment). Ken's wife, Margie, began a walking program more than 30 years ago that she still does today. She had good knowledge and good commitment but because of a very busy lifestyle needed to find the right time to exercise. She began walking the golf course near their home with three friends every morning at 6:00, and she is still walking with the same group after 30 years every Monday, Wednesday, and Friday. Admittedly, if she didn't have her group providing her with the S3—Supporting style she needed, it would have been easy to find an excuse not to walk; but when others are relying on you, you show up or you feel you are letting down the group.

After reading the first draft of this book, our publisher, Steve Piersanti, told Ken and me a similar story involving himself. At age 60, Steve is very health conscious, but because of a busy work schedule he finds it difficult to find time to exercise. He loves to play basketball, so for many years he has played pickup games with a group of young men each Tuesday and Thursday night in the gym at his church. As the organizer of the basketball games, Steve is the one with the key to open the gym and is responsible for care of the gym. Most Tuesday and Thursday nights, he has lots of excuses for not playing basketball—especially projects he is working overtime on, such as reviewing manuscripts—but he knows that if he does not show up to open the gym, he'll be letting the other players down. So Steve finds a way to participate even though he is busy or tired. After playing, he is always glad that he did, because he feels great. Steve confides that he has held on to the responsibility of opening the gym because it motivates him to do what he would otherwise frequently find an excuse not to do.

These are both great examples of exercise-minded people who achieved fitness by tying themselves to a reliable support group.

Example of a D4—Self-Reliant Achiever (High Competence/High Commitment): A good friend of mine from West Point is still an exercise fanatic at age 70. Between being a West Point graduate and serving 30 years in the army, Jim is an excellent example of fitness for his age. Without question, he is a D4 at fitness and still works out two hours per day. Because he wants to make the best use of his time and improve efficiency, he meets with me twice a year to "tune up" his program and get the latest fitness tips.

Tips for Getting Fit on a Budget

Not everyone has the luxury of joining a high-end program, so here are some tips for using your resources efficiently and budgeting for the things that are important.

- You may not need a trainer full-time, but it's a good idea to find one to set up your initial program and meet with you perhaps once a month. This way you will have a program that is customized to your needs and a professional who will help keep you accountable.

- Many large fitness clubs today sell memberships for as low as $9.99 per month. While you may not get the professional help you need at that price, most places have great equipment and a variety of exercise classes. Many of these classes build camaraderie, which can provide extra support.

- If you are not a "club person" and like to walk, consider buying a pedometer—a device that clips to your belt and counts the number of steps you take per day. It's an amazing visual motivator and costs only about $20. If you own a smartphone, numerous apps are available—many free of charge—that offer fitness tools that can turn your phone into a pedometer, measure progress toward goals, keep track of workouts, and more. Some apps even have a voice that reminds you when it's time to exercise!

- Some people prefer to work out at home. A home gym can range from an exercise mat, an exercise ball, a few sets of hand weights, and a stationary bike to a home version multistation gym, a treadmill, and an elliptical cross-trainer. The former is a $300 to $500 investment, and the latter is more like $3,000 to $5,000. A word of caution: Unless you are truly committed to your fitness program, there is a risk that this equipment will turn into expensive clothing racks!

I recall doing a home consultation for a wealthy bachelor that began with a chat in his living room. I asked him if he had any equipment. He said he did and then described all of the equipment in the last scenario. He asked me if that was good. I replied that it was, but that in many cases such machines become great racks for holding coats, ties, shirts, belts, and jackets. He had a big grin on his face and when I walked into his workout room, sure enough, everything was exactly as I had described, down to the ties and belts. We had a good laugh and then we got serious. So remember—home gym equipment is only as good as the sincerity of your motivation. If this approach interests you, a huge inventory of used equipment is available every day at bargain prices on www.craigslist.org.

- Group training sessions are an excellent way to get a lot of bang for your buck. Three to 10 people get together for a joint session with a personal trainer. This is frequently referred to as a "boot camp." The typical cost is between $5 and $20 per session. Some health care insurance providers offer discounts and, in some cases, free classes and visits to health clubs in your area. Check with your insurance company.

- Look into low-cost fitness classes, lectures, or workshops through your city or county parks and recreation department. Not only can you pick up valuable information, but it's a great way to meet like-minded people in your community who ultimately could become part of your support system.

We know that many people aren't able, like Ken, to hire coaches and assistants to help keep them on track. It might be easy to think *With all of those resources, how could anyone fail?* In fact, it can happen easily. People can pass the buck and make others accountable for their success. Remember—Ken had similar resources over the last 30 years and tried other fitness plans with only temporary results.

So why was it working this time? I'm certain it's because Ken was learning to be accountable to himself. Everyone willing to commit to a self-improvement plan needs to develop and attain the primary ingredient for success: personal accountability.

FOOD FOR THOUGHT

Think hard: Is your purpose based on what someone else wants you to do? Are you doing it for reasons coming from outside yourself or from within yourself? In order for this to be a "once and for all" program, you have to want it for you.

When considering your budget, which of the following potential expenses do you feel could be beneficial and worth the investment for you? Do you have any other ideas on how you can achieve your goals while working within your budget?

- Hire a personal trainer for support—either continuous or occasional.

(Continued next page)

- Purchase home gym equipment—either high-end or basic.
- Join a gym close to your home.
- Attend community fitness classes.
- Attend boot camp–type group training sessions.
- Purchase a good pair of walking shoes and walk with friends.
- Purchase a pedometer and keep track of your steps every day.

Who will you choose as a workout partner—someone who has the same goals as you and is as committed to success as you are?

Who will be on your support team that will hold you accountable? Think about people who care enough to help you keep your commitment to your commitment.

Great Beginnings: The First Quarter

Off to a Great Start

Ken: We were off and running after the evaluation process. I was excited because it was December, not February, and I had a highly committed partner in Tim. Our sessions three times a week really got me going on my strength and balance training with Tim providing an appropriate S1—Directing leadership style. He told me what to do and how to do it, and closely supervised my performance. With my flexibility, I was a D2—disillusioned learner, so Tim provided the S2—Coaching style I needed, with lots of direction and support. I looked forward to being around Tim. Besides being an expert in the field, he's a fun guy. His studio is only a couple of miles from our house, so it's really convenient. The time to drive back and forth, plus our session, takes less than an hour.

Having Tim work on my flexibility and balance, in addition to strength training, really helped. In addition, I went to the Egoscue clinic. Since I hadn't been there in a while, they started me off with an evaluation.

They take pictures of clients from the front, back, and both sides and that way can tell if and how a client is out of alignment—which has a lot to do with flexibility and balance. Based on that analysis, they give you an S1—Directing style menu with a series of yoga-like exercises for you to do to regain alignment. For years, the Egoscue Method® was key in saving Jack Nicklaus's back.

My son Scott was rear-ended by a car going 55 miles an hour a number of years ago. Doctors said he needed back surgery but he did Egoscue instead. He has been religious about doing his exercises ever since and has had few problems.

The problem for me was that I wasn't yet motivated to do the Egoscue stretches on my own without close supervision. Why? Because they were hard! And hard wasn't fun. I just wasn't ready to handle an S4—Delegating leadership style. Initially, it works best if you go to the clinic to do your exercises under the watchful S2—Coaching eyes of their supportive staff. Unfortunately, the clinic is 25 minutes from our place, so going for a supervised one-on-one session takes two hours, and that's hard to fit into my schedule.

For that reason, I took my assistant Mike Ortmeier with me to learn my menu so he could give me the appropriate S2—Coaching style at home. When he was with me, I did my exercises. When he wasn't, I didn't. I realized Mike and I needed to work out a clear routine if I wanted to add Egoscue to the flexibility work I was doing with Tim.

In terms of my aerobic exercise, I bought a recumbent bike. I found that it was perfect for me because it didn't hurt my back or legs the way trying to walk briskly for a couple of miles did. I wanted to build up to walking again, though, because I had set a goal for the following summer that when we got to our family's cottage in upstate New York, I wanted to walk the dirt and gravel lane going from the cottage to the main road and back. It's so beautiful there, and a round trip is about two miles.

Since Tim couldn't be with me every minute to provide the S2—Coaching supervision I needed to motivate me at home, I provided two structures of my own. First, I tried to schedule several weekly early-morning telephone calls during my workout time so I could get on the bike, put my phone on speaker, and kill two birds with one stone. When I didn't have a call, my second strategy was to watch sports on ESPN. I needed something additional to do while I was on the bike; otherwise, it got boring. Doing two 15-minute sessions a day—one in the morning and one at night—was easy. It was initially a little push to increase it to 30 minutes in one exercise period.

In regard to nutrition and weight control, another D2—disillusioned learner area for me, I benefited from two sources. As Tim mentioned, the nutrition advisor in Dr. Rice's office, Sabrina Zaslov, was helpful. To provide the direction I needed, she developed a daily menu with healthy choices I liked for breakfast, lunch, and dinner, as well as snacks. I remember hearing a speaker at a conference say that when it comes to breakfast, lunch, and dinner, most of us choose between three options for each meal. He said the key to losing weight was to find three *healthy* options for each of those meals.

To reinforce Sabrina's direction and also provide the support I needed, I rejoined Weight Watchers. Even though I was following Sabrina's plan more than theirs, I liked to go to the meetings. The groups are typically about 95 percent women, and every time you lose another five pounds, you get a star and a big hand from the group. As a person who likes to get caught doing things right, I love that reinforcement. While I have been enthusiastic about Weight Watchers in the past, my pattern had always been to go for a while and then get busy and drop out. Then I would join again and follow the same pattern. But with their great instructor Marie, who had done a program at our company, with Tim and Sabrina leading the way, and with encouragement from Margie, Scott, the rest of my family (including the famous Joy), and my work colleagues, I believed I'd be able to hang in there with Weight Watchers even through the holidays.

At the end of December, Margie and I decided to go to Rancho La Puerta Spa just across the border in Tecate, Mexico. It was a great way to top off that first month as well as to make sure that the new year got off to a good start on my fitness journey. We stayed in a cabin that was about a half mile from the dining hall and the main fitness facilities. It was a real S2—Coaching environment. Every day I did a session on the recumbent bike along with others who also weren't in top shape, and I also worked out almost every day with a member of the staff, Manny Hernandez, on strength, flexibility, and balance training. In addition, I had some sessions with a fabulous Feldenkrais teacher, Donna Wood, who was a miracle worker with flexibility. In terms of eating, it was impossible to get myself in trouble. All the food was high nutrition, low calorie, and delicious. There was no diet soda or booze except on New Year's Eve, when we were offered a glass of wine.

FOOD FOR THOUGHT

Have you ever had a hard time sticking to a fitness plan during the holiday season? What could you commit to doing differently this time that would make it less difficult?

Think of three healthy options you could choose for each meal:

- Breakfast
- Lunch
- Dinner

The Journey Begins

Tim: The evaluation process was completed by the first week of December, and we began our formal workouts at that time. We had a good fitness baseline going from the first month. Ken had been doing his aerobic exercise on his exercise bike at home for 15 minutes at a time, twice a day, five days per week. We were using the appropriate S1—Directing and S2—Coaching styles to do formal workouts together on strength, flexibility, and balance training three times per week for one hour. I had Ken increase his aerobic exercise to six days per week, integrating some interval work where he would pedal faster for one minute out of every five. Gradually he began to work on his exercise bike for 30 minutes once a day. I began adding more free weight exercises for the upper body and he progressed to doing his abdominal crunches and back extensions on the BOSU ball instead of the exercise bench.

The first three weeks of Ken's training program went very well—we even worked out on Christmas Eve morning! Ken said he was starting to feel better and his clothes were already beginning to get loose. This was the feedback I'd been hoping for.

Ever since I started my fitness business in 1986, I have always taken great care not to set false expectations. I would always laugh to myself when a 70-year-old man who had never worked out before would say, "Now, I don't want to end up built like Arnold Schwarzenegger." I would respond with glee: "That will not be a problem."

Most people I've worked with have had goals centered around weight loss. My initial promise typically has been that if they begin to exercise regularly, by the end of the first month they would be feeling better and lose some weight. However, in most cases without a dietary weight loss program, the loss of scale pounds would be very slow. I weighed Ken at 232 pounds when we started the program, and four weeks later he weighed in at Weight Watchers at 224. During the first month, I reinforced his Weight Watchers experience by encouraging him to make conscientious changes such as cutting out sweets and refined sugar, not missing meals, eating smaller portions of food, and letting exercise help metabolize the natural sugar he was ingesting.

As Ken mentioned, on the day after Christmas, he and Margie went to a health spa for a week. I knew that Ken would be getting a great education and hoped that he would get motivated to make those necessary lifestyle changes. I was also aware that he would be working with fitness trainers so, as Ken's primary coach, I sent a sheet for him to share with the staff that summarized what we were doing, and I requested that they not vary his program too much.

Ken returned at the end of the week highly energized, motivated, and down another four pounds. This was a great way to start the New Year—inspired to honor his new commitment.

FOOD FOR THOUGHT

Can you think of fun and interesting ways you could kick-start your fitness program—either alone or with someone else?

How could your support group help you keep your commitment to your commitment through a challenging time of year such as the holiday season?

Starting My Day Slowly

Ken: I was thrilled with December. When I weighed in at Weight Watchers on the Saturday following our return from Rancho La Puerta, I had lost 12 pounds. I realize that's a lot of weight to lose in just five weeks, so I tried to be realistic as I moved into the last two months of the quarter. But I even surprised myself when I lost another five pounds by the end of January. Hearing applause from my Weight Watchers friends was fun. I continuously tried to remember the great advice of the staff member at the health spa who emphasized:

You should concentrate not on *losing weight* but on *gaining health* (or, in my case, regaining fitness).

I definitely felt myself regaining fitness because of my work on the recumbent bike in the morning and my sessions with Tim. The emphasis on aerobic exercise, strength, flexibility, and balance training—combined with watching my eating and sleeping well—was a winning combination.

I also found I was really enjoying the time on my recumbent bike. To help myself move to a D3—capable but cautious performer on aerobic exercise, I made a New Year's resolution to use the bike as a way to enter my day slowly. The idea about entering my day slowly came from my friend and coauthor Jim Ballard. For years, Jim went jogging every morning. People would ask him, "How far do you go?"

Jim would reply, "I don't know."

"How long do you run?" they'd ask.

"I don't know," he'd say. "My running isn't about getting anywhere. It's the way I choose to enter my day."

What a great philosophy.

I also learned about entering my day slowly from Norman Vincent Peale, my coauthor on the book *The Power of Ethical Management*. Norman contended that we all have two selves. One is an external, task-oriented self that focuses on getting jobs done. The other is an internal, thoughtful, reflective self. The question Norman always posed was "Which self wakes up first in the morning?"

The answer, of course, is that our external, task-oriented self wakes up first. The alarm clock goes off. Have you ever thought what an awful term that is—the *alarm clock*? I once heard my friend, pastor John Ortberg, wonder, "Why isn't it the *opportunity* clock? Or the *it's going to be a great day* clock? No, it's the ALARM clock!"

So, the alarm goes off and you leap out of bed and you're into your task-oriented self. You're trying to eat while you're washing, and you're checking your e-mail as you get dressed. Then you jump in the car and you're on your speaker phone while you're driving. Next, you're going to this meeting and that meeting and running from here to there. Finally, you get home at eight or nine at night. You're absolutely exhausted, so when you fall into bed you don't even have energy to say goodnight to someone who might be lying next to you. And the next morning—*bang!*—the alarm goes off and you're at it again. Pretty soon you're in a rat race. And, as the great Hollywood philosopher Lily Tomlin once said:

"The problem with a rat race is that even if you win it, you're still a rat."

I think too often in life we're caught in an activity rat race. What we all have to do is find a way to enter our day slowly, so we can awaken our thoughtful, reflective self first in the morning. This is something I've been working on for years.

What I finally decided to do was to put a journal together with my favorite inspirational quotes from the Bible and other sources. On days when I didn't have to be on an early-morning phone call while I was on my bike, I would read my journal. It takes about 30 minutes to read my journal and reflect on what I have written. It helps the time fly, but it also helps me enter my day slowly.

The first part of my journal contains favorite Bible quotes, my personal mission statement, and other gentle reminders for the day.

The last part of what I read focuses on my health and fitness. I hope if I read it in the morning, it will guide my behavior during the day. At the top of that section it says *I am a mean and lean 185-pound golfing machine.* This has been an unfulfilled goal of mine for a long time. Let me share some of what I read from this section: My favorite Bible quote about health comes from Matthew 6:25–27, 33:

> Therefore I tell you, do not worry about your life, what you will eat or drink, or about your body or what you will wear. Is not life more important than clothes? Look at the birds of the air. They do not sow or reap or store away in barns, and yet your heavenly Father feeds them. Are you not much more valuable than they? Who of you by worrying can add a single hour to his life?
>
> So do not worry, saying, What shall we drink? or, What shall we wear? For the pagans run after all these things and your heavenly Father knows that you need them. But seek first His kingdom and His righteousness, and all these things will be given to you as well.

After reading from Matthew, I like to read two quotes from the book *Thin Within* by Judy and Arthur Halliday (2002):

> God's love for us is not based on whether we are thin, thick, tall, short, or whether or not we are in shape. But He has a plan for our body and health and we need to trust Him as our health partner. If we allow the Lord to

meet our needs, we will find the fulfillment we never knew existed and will obtain the bodies and health He wants us to have.

I believe, Lord, that You have plans for me. I believe that Your plans are not to harm me but to give me hope and a future. Lord, I thank You that Your plan isn't a diet, but a way of life in which I am no longer anxious about food or exercise. Where I begin to trust the body You have designed for me. I put my trust in You and will follow the leading of the spirit within. I choose to believe You, Lord. In His name I pray. Amen.

My friend, BJ Gallagher, wrote a wonderful book that says it all in the title: *If God Is Your Co-Pilot, Switch Seats* (2011). Always remember who is in charge—and, in my case, my ultimate health partner. These quotations might make you think that all you have to do is turn your health over to God and everything will work out. Norman Vincent Peale told me that was what a lot of people thought about the advice in his classic book *The Power of Positive Thinking* (1952)—all you had to do was think positively and everything would work out. "Not so," said Norman. "You have to do something."

Norman's favorite story to illustrate your role in life tracked a man who prayed every day to God to help him win the lottery. One night, after six months of religiously making that request and winning nothing, the man went to his prayers angry with God. He said, "Good Lord, I can't understand what's going on. I've prayed every day to you for six months to win the lottery. I'm a good man of faith, I take care of my family, and yet I've won nothing."

With that, there was a stroke of lightning and a clap of thunder. A booming voice said, "Do me a favor. Buy a ticket."

So while I believe it's good to have the Lord on your side and be positive, I also believe action is necessary.

My doctor, Lee Rice, also sees a spiritual component in the dedicated pursuit of health and fitness. He describes it this way: "In the end, fitness is a spiritual quest with meaning far beyond the numbers—it is part of becoming fully actualized as one's best self. We have been blessed with a gift of this miraculous body that requires nourishing to function at its peak effectiveness. If we truly feel blessed for the gift of life, it is then incumbent upon us to respect that gift by returning to life all of our possible talents. To the degree that we are healthy and fit—body, mind, and spirit—we are able to fully offer our gifts and talents to the world. Anything that compromises our health detracts from our ability to honor those gifts. I like the words of the late cardiologist George Sheehan: 'We are all unique, never-to-be-repeated *experiments of one* in life.'"

With the thought of honoring this body I have been given, I like to read the *Thin Within* philosophy of eating, which encourages us to be present, centered, and balanced. To reach that state, the Hallidays make the following recommendations, which I have personalized:

1. Eat only when my body is hungry.
2. Eat only when I am sitting down.
3. Eat only when my body and mind are relaxed.
4. Eat and drink what I enjoy.
5. Pay attention to my food while I am eating.
6. Eat slowly and savor each bite.
7. Stop when I am full.

After reading these recommendations, I read the seven healthy habits that Dee Edington, Margie, and I wrote about in *The One Minute Manager Balances Work and Life* (originally entitled *The One Minute Manager Gets Fit*):

1. I do not smoke.
2. I am a moderate drinker.
3. I am within five pounds of my ideal weight.
4. I am a healthy snacker.
5. I eat breakfast every day.
6. I exercise every day, or at least four times a week, for 30 minutes.
7. I sleep six to eight hours a night and wake up refreshed.

My focus during my fitness journey has been on healthy habits 3, 4, and 6—weight, snacking, and exercising. With the other four, I'm in pretty good shape: I'm a D4—self-reliant achiever.

The last piece I love to read is called "Life Abundant" in *The Wellness Book* by Donald Ardell (1996), which my daughter Debbie gave me years ago:

I want to do more than cope; I want to thrive. So I manage my stress.

I want to do more than make it through the day; I want to be energetic. So I eat nutritious food.

I want to do more than sit; I want to run. So I exercise.

I want to do more than search for happiness; I want peace. So I pray.

I want to do more than survive; I want to live. So I laugh and cry.

I want more than life, I want LIFE ABUNDANT.

Making reading my journal a major activity while on my recumbent bike helps me keep to my commitment to do aerobic exercise at least four or five times a week.

Because December and January are the lightest months for my travel, those two months were ideal for getting my fitness journey started. When I began to travel in February, it became clear that staying on my program while I was on the road would be a challenge. First, I would miss my workouts with Tim. He convinced me, though, that I should be able to hold my progress on strength training and balance. With flexibility, he thought it would be good to do my Egoscue menu, but I still was a D2—disillusioned learner on those exercises. It disappointed me, but it was the truth. With eating, I had to mentally plan ahead for each day. I was excited about my weight control progress so I was doing pretty well there.

Then a major hiccup occurred that could have side-tracked my whole program.

I was away the first week of February on business and returned with a bad cold. When it didn't seem to go away, I went to see Dr. Rice and he said one of those words nobody wants to hear: *pneumonia*. It was like a kick in the stomach. A friend who was trying to cheer me up told me, "It's God's way of saying you should slow down."

If this had been my normal starting time with Tim, I'm sure my program would have ended quickly, as usual. Believe me, I was tempted to give up! But with Joy licking my face, two good months behind me, and Tim providing the appropriate leadership style, I was determined to recover as soon as possible and get back on the program.

Even with my positive attitude, a further complication was that Tim was leaving for three weeks at the end of February to visit his daughter and her husband in Korea. While we got in a couple of light sessions before his departure, Tim suggested that Mike come to the studio with me so he could learn how to use the equipment. That way, we could keep up the strength, flexibility, and balance work while Tim and his wife Sharon were gone.

I missed a couple of Weight Watchers meetings while I was recovering from pneumonia. When I did catch one at the end of the month, I had lost three more pounds. Losing 17 pounds in three months wasn't half bad. I didn't know how to measure it, but I knew I had started to regain my fitness, even after a bout of pneumonia.

FOOD FOR THOUGHT

How do you feel about focusing more on gaining health and fitness and not so much on losing weight?

Have you ever made a conscious effort to enter your day slowly? If not, think of how you would go about it: reading something inspirational, meditating, taking a walk, or something else?

Have you ever suffered a serious health setback while in the middle of a fitness renewal? Were you able to stick to your program?

Despite a Setback, the First
Quarter Ends Well

Tim: January started out with a loud bang. After only about six weeks, Ken was down 12 pounds. It was especially impressive that he had made significant progress through the holidays.

We got in 11 formal training sessions in January. At the end of January, Ken weighed in at Weight Watchers at 215. He was doing the aerobic sessions at home on his recumbent bike—30 minutes every morning while talking on the phone, watching ESPN, or reading from his journal. Ken was still very motivated and working hard. There was no doubt in my mind that he was increasing his development level in every aspect of his program.

February was the month Ken usually began his annual two-month program. But this time when February came around, we were already two months into the program—and Ken was making great progress. I was pleased. As Ken mentioned, he was away the first week of February and returned from his trip with a bad cold, saying he didn't feel like working out. I thought he was wimping out on me, but then I found out he had pneumonia. A more compassionate trainer would have shown him some mercy! Fortunately, he wasn't hospitalized, but his doctor did order bed rest for a couple of weeks.

At this point, I became very concerned. I knew Ken would miss two weeks of exercise while recovering, and then on February 24 I was leaving the country for three weeks to visit my daughter and her husband in Korea. Missing two weeks wouldn't be too bad, but not working out for over a month could be a major setback.

I knew Ken needed a good substitute to keep our program going since he wasn't a D4—self-reliant achiever yet, so I suggested his personal assistant, Mike Ortmeier. Mike turned out to be the perfect stand-in because he was a fitness buff himself.

PRINCIPLE 5
Set Up a Support System to Hold You Accountable

I was amazed that Ken wanted to get back to our workouts as soon as he began to feel better. We got in two workouts before I left, so I was able to get Mike set up with the program at my facility. I then met with Martha Lawrence, Ken's executive editor and a successful author herself, and Renee Broadwell, who also is on Ken's editorial team and would be working directly with us on our manuscript. I told them I felt that I needed to solicit some support from within the company to keep Ken on track during my absence. They said, "No problem," and had Ken report to them weekly with a progress update.

FOOD FOR THOUGHT

Make a list of everyone, near and far, who could
   be part of your support system. Include work
   colleagues, neighbors, family, and friends you see
   often, but don't forget loved ones in other parts
   of the country or the world that you keep in touch
   with via e-mail, Internet, or phone.

When your workout partner isn't available, who could
   be an alternate person who is willing to take over
   as your key support person on a temporary basis?

Dealing with Adversity: The Second Quarter

A New Perspective—and an Unwelcome Diagnosis

Ken: March went well as Mike and I continued my training at Tim's facility. We even got in some Egoscue sessions. I didn't have a big weight loss month, but I did shed a few more pounds.

My April schedule, which included several speaking engagements in Hawaii, was a nice interruption. I took Margie, our daughter Debbie, and her almost-six-year-old son Alec with me. I love Hawaii. In fact, I can never remember having a bad time there—particularly Maui, which is where we went. Knowing that it would be a challenge to keep up my program, I worked with a coach at the hotel three times on strength, flexibility, balance, and aerobics. I got on the bike a couple of additional times and we also did a lot of walking, so I was proud of myself. I also reconnected with Alison Miller, a family friend who is a life coach in Maui. Alison came to our hotel and spent some time with us. She also does massage.

After spending time with Alison and listening to her philosophies on health, I asked her if we could talk on the phone once in a while so I could seek her advice. She gave me a group of nine stretches to do every day when I woke up. I did them religiously when I got up in the morning and continued them after I returned home. Talking with her on the phone periodically was very helpful. Alison has a natural S2—Coaching leadership style and helped me analyze what was going well and what wasn't. I realized that when I got into a busy week, unless I scheduled exercise time and said, "This is part of my schedule," I tended not to get it done. So I was really getting a lot better about putting exercise into my schedule.

In terms of my eating, I struggled a bit, because when I was in Hawaii, they had piña coladas everywhere, and I just love those. So I drank one or two piña coladas a day and I'd also let myself have dessert every once in a while. Bad boy. Oh, the guilt! Nutrition-wise, I knew I was not doing well. So when I got back home, I really concentrated on eating right for the rest of the month. When I finally did weigh myself—I avoid the scale when I think it might give me bad news—I was back down to where I wanted to be. I was even below the lowest weight I had been at Weight Watchers since I started our program.

I felt like I was coming along even with a hiccup or two and the piña colada gods tempting me. I just had to stay with it and realize that I had to take everything one day at a time. I hated to admit it, but it was taking a whole community to pull this off. In addition to Tim, Mike, my family, Joy, and my work colleagues, I now had Alison to offer encouragement periodically. My executive assistant, Margery Allen, watched my schedule like a hawk so I would have time for fitness-related activities, and Martha and Renee, my writing buddies, cheered me on.

I realize that I am fortunate to have the resources to bring together such a great team. But if I hadn't had that advantage, I believe I would have gathered friends and acquaintances who cared about me who also were interested in diet and exercise. Together we would educate ourselves and then partner to reach our fitness goals. In any case, I knew I couldn't have made it on my own. An S4—Delegating style would be a disaster. Now more than ever, I realize:

Regaining fitness is more about the journey than the announced destination.

I can see why it would be easy for anyone to relapse. For example, I went on a weekend couples retreat with Margie, and there was candy all over the place! I was pretty good about avoiding the candy, but I did have a couple of cinnamon buns. It's a constant battle to be aware of what you're doing, particularly if you have a "locked in a delicatessen overnight" mentality. If you trip, get back in step as soon as possible. That's important, because I was getting so many "You're looking good" comments, I wanted to make sure they didn't demotivate me and make me think I could relax as if I'd accomplished my goal. It's all about keeping on keeping on.

May was the best of times and the worst of times. It started off with a great relearning. Tim had told me from the beginning that to maintain a fitness regime over time, the real motivation was going to have to come from within myself, not from Scott, Margie, Joy, or anyone else. I had to want to do it for *me*. I knew that, and I felt I was moving in that direction. After all, I had been keeping on keeping on for five months. But the real truth about self-motivation was driven home by Dene Oliver, a member of my men's support group.

Our group has been meeting for a half day every four to six weeks, plus one retreat weekend a year, for over 15 years. Our only purpose is to help each other live the kind of lives we want to live. Dr. Rice is a member, along with two successful businessmen, several psychologists/psychiatrists, a retired doctor, and the former head of the YMCA for Southern California. It's quite a group. One of the most inspirational members of our group for years was a 98-year-old entrepreneur by the name of Pat Hyndman, who recently passed away. He was certainly one of the great motivators in my life. He was constantly growing and learning up until his last breath.

Dene, a very successful businessman, was about to celebrate his 20th year of sobriety. He's still very active in Alcoholics Anonymous (AA). When he heard me talk about improving my fitness, he jolted me when he said, "Ken, I think it's great that Scott kicked you in the tail and that Margie is concerned and that you have this dog you love. A lot of people start in AA because others push them there, too. But the people who are the most successful are the ones who finally realize that they want to do it for themselves. That's what I want for you—that you want to do it for yourself."

Coming from Dene, those words really hit home and reinforced what I had heard from Tim. It gave me a lot to think about.

So the motivation started when Scott confronted me, and then Dr. Rice, Margie, my assistant Margery, and others agreed with his analysis. Then I had the thought of missing the graduations of my grandsons and of my dog Joy looking for me after I had gone to rest. Now Dene was reinforcing what Tim had been telling me from the beginning—the real motivation would have to come from me.

That night I called Tim and said:

"I've finally got it! I want to be healthy and fit for *me*." And I emphasized the *me*.

Tim was excited because he knew that our book depended on my success. He also knew that, with my motivation finally coming from within, he could continue to make sure I got the appropriate help and leadership style for my development level on each of my fitness goals—and that combination would lead to success.

Then came more bad news: I was diagnosed with prostate cancer. I thought, *That's all I need. The "C" word is 10 times worse to hear than the word* pneumonia. My mind immediately went to a prostate operation. But as I learned from both Dr. Rice and my friend Dan Epstein—a member of my men's support group who had successfully overcome prostate cancer—70 percent of men get diagnosed with prostate cancer in their lives, but fewer than 10 percent ever die from it. Dan got me in touch with Dr. Mark Moyad from the University of Michigan, arguably the best prostate diagnostician in the country. He looked over all my tests, including one my father once called "the silver bugle," and felt I was a "wait and see" guy.

That was a great relief. Now I could get back to focusing on my fitness. So while May had its ups and a big down, it ended well. The first six months were successfully behind me.

FOOD FOR THOUGHT

Do you, like Ken, "avoid the scale" when you think it will give you bad news? Or do you use it as a frequent reminder to keep your commitment to your commitment?

Do you exercise while you are on vacation? If you don't stay at a hotel that has a fitness area, perhaps you could scope out a walking route nearby. Many vacation spots have other physical activities available you can do with others, such as bicycle rentals, water sports, and hiking trails.

Overcoming Obstacles

Tim: If Ken and I could keep things going this quarter, chances were good that our program would be successful. They say it takes 21 days to break an old habit—and Ken had lasted a lot longer than that.

I missed the early part of March but was glad to learn that Ken and Mike had done nine formal workout sessions during the 20 days I was away. I knew it was important to hold Ken accountable during my absence, and I believed the best way to do this was to have a formal workout schedule written out for Mike. This would ensure that each workout would be recorded so I would know what Ken did and when he did it. Mike did a great job of making sure Ken didn't miss any workouts. Better yet, Ken was happy. I was actually a little worried about getting fired—particularly when Ken called me "Mike" upon my return!

Ken and I resumed our workouts on March 18. I was impressed that his attitude was still very positive. It would have been easy for him to get discouraged and quit with a setback like pneumonia, particularly when he might have lost some strength and gained a few pounds due to inactivity. However, I was pleased to see that he had regained any strength he'd lost and, amazingly, he was down a few more pounds. So March ended well. There's an important lesson to be learned here:

When you have a setback, take time out to recover, and then resume your program.

April brought some important breakthroughs for Ken. He took a week-long trip to Hawaii and immediately went into a vacation mode of "When in Rome, do as the Romans do." However, he must have realized the importance of continuing to exercise because he worked with a trainer for three sessions while he was there. Although Ken was working hard at the gym in Hawaii, he started eating and drinking a little carelessly. Then he visited with an old friend and life coach, Alison Miller, who saw that he was starting to slip and immediately helped him get back on track. Also, he got enough "You're looking good" comments to keep him going forward.

Upon his return, he called me right away and we got right back to work. The rest of April went well. It seemed that Ken finally understood how important it was to keep on keeping on and not revert back to old behaviors. The key to this change in attitude was that Ken's motivation now was to work on regaining his fitness for himself rather than for Scott, Margie, Joy, or anyone else. This point was driven home by his friend who was celebrating his 20th anniversary of sobriety. What a blessing!

As we were busy patting ourselves on the back, another obstacle appeared: Ken was diagnosed with prostate cancer in the middle of May. All of a sudden, our number one priority was Ken's health and well-being. We immediately turned our focus to how he could best deal with this diagnosis.

Thankfully, tests revealed that Ken's prostate cancer was in the very early stages and did not require radical treatment. Dr. Rice assembled the best team of physicians and they decided to watch it. In the meantime, exercise would play a vital role in maintaining Ken's health. A healthy diet was also a key player. To my great pleasure, Ken—a real fighter—said, "Let's get back to work and beat this thing." With that, we continued with his program—full steam ahead.

This all served to remind both of us that Ken's journey wasn't a one-year plan but rather a *lifetime* plan.

PRINCIPLE 6
Have Measurable Milestones to Stay Motivated

I thought it would be useful to do a midterm evaluation to see how Ken was progressing, so May concluded with a fitness evaluation—because on any journey, it is very important to have milestones. I also felt an evaluation at this time was important to keep Ken motivated. I knew he had made great progress, and I wanted to show him how well he had done. I began to worry that Ken might think *What kind of training program am I on? I'm supposed to be doing this to improve my fitness, and in six months I get pneumonia and am diagnosed with prostate cancer!* Fortunately, Ken is a realist. The program was progressing with real life plugged in.

The Midterm Evaluation

I began Ken's exam with the easiest measurement: body weight. This simply involved reading the scale. In six months, Ken's weight had dropped from 232 to 212. A loss of 20 pounds equaled an average of just under one pound per week. When weight is lost by diet alone and no exercise, part of that loss is muscle tissue, which is not desirable. My objective with Ken was to gain muscle tissue and lose body fat only. Because his strength had increased considerably, he actually gained some muscle weight, so the actual fat loss may have been even greater. There are numerous methods for measuring body fat, ranging from skin-fold thickness to bio-impedance. In my opinion, most of these tests are unreliable. I believe the most significant outcome has to do with reshaping the body to the desirable goal. Ken's objective measurements were as follows:

Weight: minus 20 pounds
Height: no difference
Neck: minus 0.5 inch
Chest (relaxed): minus 1 inch
Chest (expanded): no difference
Waist: minus 2 inches

Hips: minus 1.5 inches
Bicep (relaxed): minus 0.5 inch
Bicep (flexed): minus 0.5 inch
Thigh—R: minus 1 inch
Thigh—L: no difference
Balance on left foot: plus 15 seconds
Balance on right foot: plus 18 seconds
Stand on BOSU: plus 35 seconds
Hamstring flex—R: improved 12 degrees
Hamstring flex—L: improved 13 degrees
Heel cord—R: improved 6 degrees
Heel cord—L: improved 4 degrees

Ken's clothes no longer fit correctly—they were getting loose. Darn, he had to get a new wardrobe! Ken was feeling better, moving easier, getting lots of compliments, and, most important, feeling good about himself.

FOOD FOR THOUGHT

What two or three milestones can you use during the course of your fitness program that will help you measure your progress?

How can your own internal motivation help when you are confronted by temptation in the form of sweets, high-calorie drinks, or other obstacles that stand in the way of your goals?

Heading into Summer: The Third Quarter

My 50-Year Class Reunion and Summer Retreat

Ken: I look forward to June every year, but this June was especially sweet because it started out with my 50th reunion at Cornell. Margie and I both graduated from Cornell—she was a year behind me—so we developed many good Cornell friendships together. The reunion was a great excuse to get together with this group as well as a lot of other good people.

It was hard to imagine that 50 years had gone by since we graduated. Tim and I have mentioned a few times that I was starting to get a number of "You're looking good" comments. That phrase was originated by Frank Rhodes, who was president of Cornell when I was getting my doctorate. Frank used to say, "There are three stages of life: youth, adulthood, and 'You're looking good.'" At the opening cocktail party, just for the fun of it, Margie and I went in different directions to see how many "You're looking good" comments we would get. After about a half hour, we found each other and compared notes. I beat her by one—I had eight "You're looking good" comments to Margie's seven. So for me, that was an important mission accomplished. The reunion was a ball. I probably drank a little too much beer, but I was grateful to be alive and getting more fit week by week and month by month.

Traditions and Temptations at a Special Summer Place

After the Cornell reunion, we returned to San Diego for a couple of weeks before we headed back to upstate New York and Skaneateles Lake for the summer. *Skaneateles* is an Iroquois term that means long, narrow lake, which describes it perfectly—it's 17 miles long and about three-quarters of a mile wide. Our cottage on the lake is 45 minutes from Cornell.

When Margie's mom, Natalie, was in college, she had a roommate whose family had a place on Skaneateles Lake. After Natalie and her husband Red made a few visits there, they fell in love with Skaneateles. In 1946, they bought 280 feet of lakefront for $300 from a farmer's widow. Quite a deal! So Margie has been going to the lake during the summer since she was six years old.

Spending summers in Skaneateles has been a tradition for us ever since Margie and I got married in June 1962. When we were graduate students or members of the faculty or staff at universities, it was easy to justify. After all, our cottage was a great place to do research and writing, particularly with the Cornell library nearby. Going to Skaneateles in the summer became a way of life. So when we started our company in 1979 in Escondido, California, we told our first colleagues, "By the way, we won't be here in July or August, so you'll have to get along without us." Each year, everyone still says good-bye to us at an all-company meeting in June and then welcomes us back in September.

While we engage in all kinds of outside activities at the lake, eating and drinking and making merry are central during our time there. Family and friends are coming and going. It's a special place to visit for a lot of the important people in our lives.

Realizing I still wasn't a D4—self-reliant achiever in terms of my fitness program, I took two precautions to make sure my efforts did not head south in the summer. First, I invited Mike Ortmeier to spend a good part of the summer with us since his wife, Dorothy, was away for extended trips to Europe and South Africa as one of our global sales associates. Mike, who has a good S2—Coaching leadership style, made sure I didn't overeat and that I got in plenty of walks and good exercise. Second, Anton Kowalski, a local fitness coach I had worked with in years past, worked me out two or three times a week at a local facility.

As a result, I came back in early September having not lost much ground on my aerobic exercise (I had bought a recumbent bike for the lake) or on my strength, flexibility, and balance training (Anton is great, and Mike was a plus, working with me on my Egoscue stretches). In terms of my nutrition and weight control, Alison Miller, who was spending time back east seeing family and friends, came for a visit. During her time at the lake, she helped me look at healthy eating choices. She even made some veggie shakes that weren't bad. I took advantage of her visit for a couple of great massages as well as extra stretching and flexibility exercises. Alison has been a great supporter of my fitness journey.

Even with all the help, I gained a few pounds by the time we got back to San Diego in early September. The corn on the cob, Italian sausages, and gin and tonics were so good! "Perfect" has never been one of my characteristics. But all in all, I felt good about the summer. I was ready to finish with a strong fall and last quarter of my yearlong journey.

FOOD FOR THOUGHT

Do you feel that it's more challenging to follow a fitness plan when you are at home or when you are away from home? Why?

What are some of your strategies for eating healthy when everyone around you is in a party mood?

Do you get down on yourself if you aren't "perfect" every day when working on a fitness program? If so, how can you snap out of that attitude?

Setting Up an Absentee Program

Tim: June is often a month for Ken to wind down from a busy spring. Then the prize of the year—summer on Skaneateles Lake in upstate New York—kicks in.

June started off with Ken feeling very good about himself as he left on a short trip to Cornell University for his 50th class reunion. When he returned, I asked him how it went. He said it was great and he got a lot of "You're looking good" comments. With that feedback, I believed that we had accomplished goal number one. The remainder of June went very well. We got in 10 good workouts, and Ken worked hard on his aerobic activity and weight control.

On June 30, Ken and the family departed for their summer cottage in Skaneateles. I stayed at home in San Diego—not a bad place to be left behind. Our separation did, however, present a significant challenge for me. Somehow I had to ensure that Ken didn't gain any weight and that he would continue his workouts while not in my presence.

The Inevitable Plateau

In terms of weight loss, during the first six months Ken was down 20 pounds on the scale. Again, his actual fat loss was more than that because he was quite a bit stronger so he had gained some muscle weight. Drawing on my many years of experience, I began preparing Ken for the upcoming, and certain, plateau. This is the time when the body is reluctant to give up too much of its stored energy (fat) and resists change—so no matter how hard you work, or how diligently you diet, you seemingly can't lose weight. In fact, sometimes you even gain back a few pounds. This can become very discouraging and is the point where many people give up. This plateau can last a while, so I wanted to be sure that Ken fully understood it before he left for the summer because he would be away from my direct involvement and on his own for two months. An important aspect of my message also had to stress that while plateauing was natural, gaining weight was to be avoided. I only hoped they didn't make piña coladas in upstate New York!

In terms of exercise, although I believed Ken had progressed from a D1 to a D3 in strength and balance training and from a D2 to a D3 in aerobic exercise and flexibility, I felt he still needed occasional S2—Coaching to monitor his progress and prevent injury. He certainly couldn't handle an S4—Delegating style yet in these areas.

Ken's plan was to work out with Anton Kowalski, a trainer he had worked with in the past in Skaneateles. I contacted Anton by phone and explained our project. He said he would be happy to keep Ken on track. I connected with Ken at least once a week. He told me that getting the workouts in was relatively easy, but the eating and drinking management was difficult because everyone was in a vacation mode. It was tough for him to watch everyone drinking their favorite drink at cocktail hour as he sipped green tea, or seeing them enjoy desserts after dinner while he'd eat a grape. Ken's assistant Mike was there much of the time, and Ken also had a visit from his friend and life coach Alison Miller. So in a sense, my substitutes were there to help Ken deal with these temptations so he could stick as close to his commitment as possible.

My primary goal was to have Ken maintain his current body weight, have formal workouts at least twice per week, and do a minimum of 30 minutes of aerobic work every day. Ken made one brief visit back to San Diego on August 24, and he and I had a workout at my facility at 6:00 that morning. I was happy to find that even though he had gained back a few pounds, he had stuck with all of the workouts. One of the goals of the long-term exercise program was to help increase his metabolism. After nine months of consistent exercise, he was seeing some of this benefit.

As you can see, even when it's not summer, Ken is often away from home on business. For those of you who share Ken's "road warrior" lifestyle, remember that when you are on the road for more than a few days, it is critically important to not only watch your food choices but also maintain some type of fitness plan. In Resources II, Tim's Toolbox, I will discuss in detail what you should consider for a traveling program.

FOOD FOR THOUGHT

If you travel for work, what do you see as the most difficult challenges to your fitness routine when you are on the road?

If you have ever hit a plateau during a weight loss program—when no matter how healthy you ate or how often you exercised you couldn't seem to make any progress—did you keep on keeping on? What did you do to help yourself through this time?

In the past have you used an event, such as a family wedding or an upcoming 10K run, as a goal for getting back in shape? Did you achieve your goal for the event? If so, did you keep in shape after the event was over?

6

The Home Stretch:
The Fourth Quarter

Finishing Strong

Ken: Because I had gained a couple of pounds over the summer, I decided I needed to do something in September to give myself a little extra boost on the nutrition and weight control part of my program. I kept hearing Ted Leitner, the radio play-by-play announcer for the San Diego Padres baseball team, talk about Medifast: "If you've been struggling to lose weight, Medifast will get you results." So not too long after we returned from Skaneateles, I thought, *Why not? Maybe it can get me over this weight plateau.*

I called Dr. Rice to get his feedback. He checked out Medifast in his circles with positive results. The combination of healthy choice meals together with prepackaged meals and snacks seemed to make sense, and these foods were nutrition balanced. I went ahead and made an appointment at a nearby location. When I went in for my appointment, the woman who ran the office gave me an overview of the Medifast system and the best strategy for me. I was impressed, so I joined. It's not cheap, but I thought it was worth it.

Although I was a big fan of my Weight Watchers group, I knew I needed closer supervision. In the Medifast program, you are assigned to a counselor who meets with you once a week, weighs you, looks over your eating diary, and works with you to develop a strategy for your next week. My counselor was a delightful woman named Jacquie Schumaker. With Jacquie I would be getting an S2—Coaching leadership style with direction and support, rather than the less intensive S3—Supporting leadership style used by Weight Watchers. It worked—and by the end of September I was down to 206. Not bad!

Another important development happened during this last quarter. I reconnected with Art Turock, author of *Getting Physical* (1988), who had taught me the difference between *interest* and *commitment.* He helps leaders develop people into elite performers. Art and I agreed to talk for 30 minutes on the phone at 7:00 a.m. every Monday or Tuesday.

You might be saying, *Okay, Blanchard. Does it really take this big a village to keep your commitment to your commitment? You keep adding people to your team.*

My response is: "Hey! When you can smell the end zone and the possibility of seeing a victory, would you not welcome a few additional blockers? Sure you would!" I wanted to finish strong.

Unfortunately, I faced a new challenge in October while playing golf in Florida as part of an annual tradition with a bunch of my Cornell buddies. We have a great time trying to beat each other. While attempting to outdrive them all with my new, powerful swing, I hit *terra firma* and ruptured my left bicep muscle. I knew I had hurt something, but being around my buddies I just took some ibuprofen and hung in there and continued playing. My classmate Dick Tatlow and I won the whole shooting match on the 18th hole, when I curled in a downhill 15-foot par putt.

After a visit to the emergency room that afternoon, I was advised to see my doctor as soon as I returned home. I decided not to play the final optional morning round in order to rest my injured arm. By the time I flew home, my entire left arm and hand were black and blue.

Back in San Diego, Dr. Rice sent me for an MRI, which revealed a rupture at the midpoint of my bicep muscle belly. At first I was very concerned. I thought, *Oh, no! This is the end of my program. How stupid!* I certainly didn't want a major setback so close to the finish line. Fortunately, it turned out that it wasn't as bad as it looked and, with Tim's prodding and Dr. Rice's consent, I was still able to work out a modified program with Tim and continue my aerobic work on my recumbent bike.

They say bad things happen in threes—so with the pneumonia, the prostate cancer diagnosis, and now my bicep muscle injury, I hoped the bad news was over. The good news is that through it all with the team I had gathered, I was able to keep on keeping on.

November brought some breakthroughs. I had to reduce my ring and watchband size and I broke the 200-pound mark. I couldn't wait to look at the comparative data that Tim was gathering for his end-of-year evaluation. Why? Because I knew it was a year when I not only lost weight but also regained my fitness.. Hallelujah! Praise the Lord, Tim, all my family including Joy, my friends, and my colleagues. I had made it!

FOOD FOR THOUGHT

Ken changed his weight loss plan when he realized he needed closer supervision. Are you getting the right leadership style for what you are trying to accomplish? When you think about the goal of weighing less, how much, if any, outside supervision do you think you will need to succeed?

Have you ever had a sports injury that kept you from your regular exercise program? Looking back, what could you have done to get back "in the groove" afterward?

New Habits Becoming a Way of Life

Tim: This was the home stretch—the final three months of our journey. It was no time to rest on our laurels. We had to keep on keeping on!

Ken resumed his workouts with me the first week of September and we began the final phase of our yearlong program. His body weight was 214, up just two pounds from when he'd left two months earlier—not bad. While he was getting a lot of "You're looking good" comments, I knew that one of his goals from the beginning was to break 200 on the scale.

As Ken mentioned, he decided that the best way to get there was to go on a diet that not only was strict but also had managed accountability. His choice was Medifast. As I have stated earlier, I am not a big believer in diets, but I did like the way Medifast integrated regular healthy meals with packaged foods. I also know that Ken works best when he has supportive supervision and accountability. This S2—Coaching style seems to work best in areas where he is struggling.

By the end of September, Ken was down to 206 and feeling great about it.

As Ken related, another important new aspect of his fitness journey occurred in the last quarter when he became reacquainted with Art Turock, an exercise/life coach he had worked with many years before. Because Art was a big advocate of Ken's keeping his commitment to his commitment, I was glad to have him on the team.

Keep in mind that even if you aren't in a position to hire a professional fitness support team:

Very few people can accomplish a major life change by themselves.

Ideally, everyone needs to have at least one or two friends or family members to be their accountability partners and help them accomplish their goals.

September ended up being a very good exercise month. Ken actually seemed to be enjoying his workouts and had an attitude of ownership of his results.

A Sports Injury

October began with yet another obstacle when Ken ruptured his left bicep muscle while playing golf with his old buddies in Florida. This was a very unusual injury. Fortunately, it wasn't a complete rupture. Ten years earlier, I had complete ruptures of both distal bicep attachments in a freak accident. This required a surgical reattachment and extensive rehab, so I personally knew what a large bullet we had dodged.

Sports and training injuries are a fact of life. Any time you put added stress on the body, you are subject to some kind of injury. Most training injuries are avoidable with proper preparation. Sports injuries, in contrast, occur at a very high rate. Most adult sports injuries occur during "weekend warrior" activities.

At one time, these injuries constituted the number one reason for visits to the emergency room on weekends. While there are many reasons for this, the most common cause of this type of injury is a lack of physical preparation—people think they can participate at the same level they did in high school and college. These injuries range from concussions and broken bones to skin abrasions and bruises. In Ken's case, this injury was just an unfortunate accident.

Ken's injury teaches an important lesson. When an injury occurs, the first thing to do is to confer with a doctor.

By early November, Ken's arm showed significant improvement. Because of Ken's rapid recovery, I got the green light from his doctor to work around the injury site and to do mild rehab, stretching, and friction massage on the injury itself.

When you have a muscle injury such as Ken's, it generally takes four to eight weeks to fully recover. Many people would use this as an excuse to stop working out and allow the total body to rest. A total break of a month or more could have set us back six months and made it difficult to resume the program. Fortunately, Ken was still able to continue his aerobic exercise, strength, flexibility, and balance training for three limbs and his entire torso. We were also able to do rehab on the injured limb, so once Ken had regained pain-free range of motion, he quickly recovered the strength in his injured arm.

After 11 months of training, Ken had established a very positive attitude. This, along with encouragement and the proper guidance, allowed him to overcome each of the obstacles he had faced through our time together.

On Monday, November 7, Ken came into my facility bragging about another milestone. Over the weekend he had to have his wedding ring reduced in size and two links removed from his watchband. He also reported that he was weighing 199 pounds on his home scale. We were going to make it!

As Thanksgiving approached, Ken was determined to stay with the Medifast protocol with the exception of Thanksgiving Day. At the end of November, one year from the beginning of our program, we did our official measurements. Here are the results:

ONE-YEAR REEVALUATION	Nov. 25, 2010	May 27, 2011	Nov. 26, 2011
Body weight	232 pounds	212 pounds	199 pounds
Height	68.0 inches	68.0 inches	68.5 inches
Neck	17.0 inches	16.5 inches	15.75 inches
Head from wall	3.5 inches	2.75 inches	2.0 inches
Chest (relaxed)	41.5 inches	40.5 inches	40 inches
Chest (inflated)	42 inches	42 inches	41 inches
Waist (navel level)	45 inches	43 inches	41 inches
Hips	46 inches	44.5 inches	42 inches
Bicep (relaxed)	14 inches	13.5 inches	13.25 inches
Bicep (flexed)	14 inches	13.5 inches	14 inches
Thigh—R	26 inches	25 inches	24.5 inches
Thigh—L*	24 inches	24 inches	23.5 inches
Balance on L foot	10 seconds	25 seconds	68 seconds
Balance on R foot	2 seconds	20 seconds	55 seconds
Stand on BOSU	0 seconds	35 seconds	2 minutes
Hamstring flex—R	minus 35 degrees	minus 23 degrees	minus 18 degrees
Hamstring flex—L	minus 45 degrees	minus 32 degrees	minus 23 degrees
Heel cord—R	0 degrees	minus 6 degrees	minus 8 degrees
Heel cord—L	minus 5 degrees	minus 9 degrees	minus 12 degrees

*Arthritic knee.

It's also interesting to look at the change in the numbers from Ken's examinations with Dr. Rice:

	Dec. 14, 2010	Dec. 20, 2011
Height	68.0 inches	68.5 inches
BP	116/72	112/74
Resting HR	72	60
Sit-ups	50	60
Push-ups	9	22
Total cholesterol	153	136
LDL	86	63
HDL	46	60
Cholesterol/HDL ratio	3.3	2.2
Triglycerides	107	39

Dr. Rice offered some helpful comments about Ken's improving health and fitness:

"I think Ken's numbers are spectacular! But more impressive than just the improvement in his numbers is what this means in terms of increased functionality. All of these positive changes are the cornerstones of increased engagement in life, enjoyment in daily living, appearance, self-pride, quality of life, and longevity. Especially notable is the improvement in Ken's balance and coordination, which equates to less risk of injury and increased ability to recapture his body's innate abilities. Improvement in core strength and extremity strength shows that Ken's initial test results were examples of *sarcopenia*, a condition that results from a sedentary lifestyle and can lead to premature aging and disability.

"Getting healthy and fit means so much more than looking good. A healthier adult automatically is at less risk for cardiovascular disease, stroke, dementia, erectile dysfunction, diabetes, and even all-cause mortality.

"We're all athletes. It's just that some of us are in training and some aren't!"

FOOD FOR THOUGHT

What would be the most difficult part of sustaining your commitment to your commitment once you had reached your goals?

What would be the biggest incentive for you not to slide backward once achieving your fitness goals?

The last time you reached a goal you had been trying to achieve for a long time, how did you celebrate?

7

Final Thoughts

Role Models, Cheerleaders, and Persistence

Ken: I have several pieces of advice for people like you who may be starting to work on a program to do something important for yourself that you've been putting off for a long time.

First, think about any role models who exemplify what you are trying to accomplish. Why is that important? My wife Margie has said for a long time:

"A goal is a dream with a deadline."

To me, the dream that you are attempting to make come true will be found in someone who models what you desire. Three people came to mind as health and fitness models for me at my age.

When we first came to San Diego, Margie and I were into jogging. Ed Coverly, the fellow who led our jogging group, was 65 years old and said he didn't start running until he was 60. In recent years, he was running two or three marathons a year. Now I don't want to run a marathon, but Ed comes to mind when I think of someone who got himself in really good shape after he was 60.

Norman Vincent Peale was another great example for me. I met him when he was 86 years old. I'd pick him up at the airport and say, "Norman, why don't you wait here and I'll get the car?" and he'd say, "No! I've been sitting too long. I need to take a brisk walk!" He always was within five pounds of what he weighed when he was 18 years old. Yet here he was in his late 80s saying, "Let's take a walk." Norman and his wife Ruth walked together every morning for at least two miles. They would hold hands but not talk. They called it "our alone time together." They were both models for me in terms of my ambition to make it to 95 or 100 years old and still be fit and healthy. Norman passed away at 95 and Ruth died a couple of years ago at 101. I want to grow up to be like them someday!

I already mentioned my third role model—Pat Hyndman, a member of my men's support group, who lived a full life and left us at 98. He was a lifelong learner as well as a teacher and mentor to all who knew him.

My second piece of advice is when you start a program, get some professional help as well as support from family, friends, and colleagues. As you have read, I put together quite a team besides Tim. I couldn't have accomplished my fitness goals all by myself. I suspect you may need some help, too—although maybe not as much as I did. So get your ego out of the way and realize that trying to grind it out all by yourself doesn't usually work.

One final thought: Once you feel you have reached the goals you set, don't be too quick to let the support team you've assembled off the hook. As we've said, the road to nowhere is paved with good intentions. It will take you a while before you become a true D4—self-reliant achiever who can handle an S4—Delegating leadership style on every one of your goals. For years I've been great at making announcements about getting fit, and even smart in seeking initial help. But every time I would hit D2 and become a disillusioned learner, rather than continuing to get coached, I would drop the program and not keep my commitment to my commitment to be a healthy and fit human being. So don't give up—keep it going until you can really be self-motivated.

As I write this in November 2013, it has been three full years since I started my program with Tim. While we didn't document the second or third year, I'm proud to say that my development level has improved significantly in most areas of fitness. I'm even closing in on becoming a D4—self-reliant achiever in more areas besides just my rest and sleep.

In terms of aerobic exercise, riding my recumbent bike for 30 to 45 minutes at least five times a week has become a way of life. I am becoming a D4—self-reliant achiever in this fitness area. I also achieved my goals of walking the lane at our lake cottage in upstate New York as well as the loop in our neighborhood in San Diego, which is much hillier and over two miles. Both are favorite activities for my walking partner, Joy. One of my motivations for my fitness program, to avoid knee replacement surgery, has been met with success. Because of my weight loss and increased fitness with Dr. Rice's and Tim's encouragement, such an operation is not necessary at this time.

I still see Tim two or three times a week when I'm in town, and Anton Kowalski at the lake in the summer, so they can continue working with me on my strength, flexibility, and balance. I enjoy my S3—Supporting times with them but feel it still makes sense to have supervision, S2—Coaching with my strength and balance training to prevent possible injury.

Regarding flexibility, I decided to bite the bullet and get a new menu of exercises and stretches from the Egoscue facility. I've stuck with it and it's now something I do five times a week with encouragement and cheerleading from my assistant, Mike. I am moving slowly from a D2—disillusioned learner to a D3—capable but cautious performer on flexibility. Someday I hope to be a D4—self-reliant achiever with my flexibility routines. Tim also continues to build on the flexibility I have been gaining from my Egoscue sessions.

With regard to nutrition and weight control, I haven't continued Medifast but have rejoined Weight Watchers. I've become much better at managing my own weight and nutrition program, but I still love the S3—Supporting cheerleading. I'm proud to report that as of this writing I have broken the 190-pound barrier and am now over 40 pounds lighter than when I started. I am moving closer to being able to handle an S4—Delegating style on eating.

So I am a happy camper. I know I have not only lost weight but also gained health. As a result, I am feeling better physically as well as intellectually, emotionally, and spiritually. I feel healthier, my mind is clear and sharp, I am no longer a stimulus-response machine, and I know more than ever that God is good.

In case you need a reminder, here are the six principles I lived by during my health and fitness journey. Tim and I feel that a person who adheres to all six principles will have the best chance at success in committing to a major life change such as the one I have undergone.

SIX PRINCIPLES OF A SUCCESSFUL HEALTH AND FITNESS PROGRAM

1. Have Compelling Reasons and a Purpose
2. Establish a Mutual Commitment to Success
3. Learn About Situational Leadership® II
4. Develop Age-Appropriate Goals
5. Set Up a Support System to Hold You Accountable
6. Have Measurable Milestones to Stay Motivated

I hope reading about my journey will motivate you to reexamine a goal you have been wanting to accomplish that you have been putting off. Good luck. Hang in there. Keep your commitment to your commitment—but don't do it alone. Get some help and teach your support team Situational Leadership® II. God bless.

A Successful Journey

Tim: What we have described for you in this book is Ken's successful one-year journey toward becoming more fit. It required Ken to not only change some of his old habits but also incorporate new habits into a new way of life.

With any program of this magnitude, adults need time not only for old habits to change but also for new habits to become a way of life. Ken encountered a number of obstacles during his journey but developed the attitude that they were mere setbacks. After the obstacle would pass, he would resume his program.

With a yearlong program, as we mentioned earlier, it is important to have milestones as well as specific goals. Ken's first goal was to attend his 50th class reunion at Cornell and hear his classmates say, "You're looking good." Although somewhat general in nature, these observations were very important to him. Attending that reunion, along with Margie's Cornell reunion and their 50th wedding anniversary celebration the following year, ultimately gained Ken enough "You're looking good" comments to satisfy this goal many times over.

As an educated health and fitness trainer, I would have preferred that Ken's goals were to lower his cholesterol by a specific number, reduce his blood pressure and body fat, and improve his functional fitness. The reality is, through his achievement of the outcome *he* desired, he also accomplished the end results *I* was hoping for—a true win/win.

As Ken has related, virtually every parameter of his physical fitness continues to improve. He is stronger and fitter, has reached his ultimate weight goal, and has advanced in his development level in all of his fitness areas. I still enjoy our times together as we continue with strength, flexibility, and balance training. As Ken's health and fitness keep improving, my leadership style has moved more and more to a predominantly S3—Supporting style as he continues to set new goals for himself. We will soon begin our fourth year of working together.

To illustrate that Ken's fitness program truly has become a way of life, it's a joy to show you a comparison between where Ken began three years ago, where he was after his one-year program was completed, and where he is now after three years have passed.

THREE-YEAR REEVALUATION			
	Nov. 25, 2010	Nov. 26, 2011	Nov. 25, 2013
Body weight	232 pounds	199 pounds	188.5 pounds
Height	68.0 inches	68.5 inches	68.5 inches
Neck	17.0 inches	15.75 inches	15.5 inches
Head from wall	3.5 inches	2.0 inches	1.5 inches
Chest (relaxed)	41.5 inches	40 inches	40 inches
Chest (inflated)	42 inches	41 inches	42 inches
Waist (navel level)	45 inches	41 inches	40 inches
Hips	46 inches	42 inches	41 inches
Bicep (relaxed)	14 inches	13.25 inches	13 inches
Bicep (flexed)	14 inches	14 inches	14.5 inches
Thigh—R	26 inches	24.5 inches	24 inches
Thigh—L*	24 inches	23.5 inches	23.5 inches
Balance on L foot	10 seconds	68 seconds	120 seconds
Balance on R foot	2 seconds	55 seconds	120 seconds
Stand on BOSU	0 seconds	2 minutes	Indefinitely
Hamstring flex—R	minus 35 degrees	minus 18 degrees	minus 15 degrees
Hamstring flex—L	minus 45 degrees	minus 23 degrees	minus 25 degrees
Heel cord—R	0 degrees	minus 8 degrees	minus 8 degrees
Heel cord—L	minus 5 degrees	minus 12 degrees	minus 12 degrees

*Arthritic knee.

Usually an epilogue suggests an ending—but after three years of progress, Ken's fitness journey continues to be an important part of his life. When Ken and I last met, we both put our right hands on our left shoulders and our left hands on our right shoulders and gave ourselves a hug. Then we hugged each other.

I hope Ken's story has inspired you to embark on your own journey of continuous improvement toward optimal health and fitness, or whatever goal you feel is important for your best possible quality of life. We wish you nothing but success.

RESOURCES I
Pearls of Wisdom
from the Experts

Since I love learning, I am constantly seeking the advice of experts in my field. What follows are valuable pearls of wisdom from five such experts.

—Tim Kearin

The First Pearl: Fitness and the Aging Process

Marcus Elliott, M.D., and Mike Walker

Throughout this book, reference is made to having an age-appropriate exercise program. We know that the body declines physically from maturity. I have experienced this personally in my own training and in training clients as they age, and have researched the subject extensively.

Marcus Elliott, M.D.

I thought the best way to sum up this topic would be to have a discussion with Dr. Marcus Elliott. Marcus has a medical degree from Harvard University and is an internationally recognized leader in the field of performance enhancement and the development of elite athletes. Rather than practice formal medicine, Marcus chose to use his medical training and research to develop the finest conditioning and injury prevention program available to professional athletes. The athletes he trains "age out" of his program before 40, as they are no longer physically capable of training at that level.

I asked Marcus why, with a medical degree from Harvard, he chose a career in sports conditioning rather than medicine.

He replied, "At age 16 I knew I wanted to train professional athletes. I later figured out that by going for a medical degree I would be able to get the best education available on injury prevention and on exactly how the human body functions."

Marcus has created one the nation's premier training facilities for top-level athletes, P3 in Santa Barbara, California. I told Marcus I was writing a book dealing with exercise and the aging process and was particularly interested in how aging affects training in top athletes. I believed that knowing this would give me a better idea of how to train a nonathlete.

He said, "In order to achieve optimal physical performance and to prevent injury, a top athlete has to train at a very high level of intensity. The training also includes placing great loads on the muscles and tendons to prepare them for the extreme stresses that occur in high-level physical performance. My own research indicates that even the best athletes are unable to do these workouts after about age 38. This is also why many professional athletes end their careers around that same age. The ones who continue to work out at that higher level have difficulty keeping up, don't recover as quickly, and are more prone to injury."

I asked Marcus whether athletes at that level who are extremely self-motivated still need a support system. His reply was "Yes—their support system is the athletes they train with who will not allow them to fail."

In conclusion, I asked Marcus what recommendations he would make to a middle-aged person wanting to start a serious exercise program.

He replied, "It's important that the individual outline their program with a trainer who is familiar with the individual's age group, and that the trainer matches the program to the individual's specific desires and needs. It's also extremely important that the person have a support system to ensure long-term success."

Mike Walker

To further satisfy my curiosity, I met with Mike Walker, who is not a professional athlete but a high achiever who always wanted to maintain optimal fitness. At 42 years of age, Mike is CEO of Baswood Corporation, a company that provides low-cost, environmentally friendly alternatives for biosolids and wastewater solutions for municipal and industrial clients. Mike has climbed Mount Rainier, Mount Shasta, and Tibet's Mount Kailash. He has run several marathons as well as the Himalayan 100-Mile Stage Race, a four-day race, and the Racing the Planet Gobi March, a 150-mile five-day race in the Gobi Desert.

I wanted to meet with Mike because Dr. Elliott had told me Mike was over 40 years old but insisted on working in his program with the younger high-level athletes. Mike was most gracious to consent to an informal interview.

Mike told me he played all of the major sports in high school, football at UC Berkeley, and then weekend basketball after he began his career. He said, "The reason I moved from weekend basketball to extreme endurance events was because all of the really hard-core basketball players quit playing. I wanted a great physical challenge. My deep motivation was to be the fittest I could be for my age." I asked him about his support system. He replied, "My wife not only has been a huge support; she also trained and did several of these events with me."

Mike is now training for competitive beach volleyball—and wants to be the best—so he entered Dr. Elliott's high-level athlete training. He found, however, that he could not keep up with what the other athletes were doing and had to work at an age-appropriate level of intensity. When I asked him whether his goals and motivations have changed over the years, he said that now, at age 42, he is most interested in staying fit for health reasons.

Finally, I asked Mike the same question I asked Dr. Elliott: What would he recommend to a middle-aged person wanting to begin a serious exercise program? His response was similar to that of the doctor: "Select an age-appropriate program, no matter how serious you are. Have a strong support system and have a purpose—which, at middle age and over, should be directed more toward health than anything else."

We can learn some important lessons from Dr. Elliott, a professional trainer, and Mike Walker, a nonprofessional, goal-oriented individual:

1. Find an age-appropriate program. If you don't want to spend the money on a full-time coach, find a trainer familiar with your age group who can at least set up your program.

2. Have a support system of individuals who will stand by you in good times and tough times.

3. Have a distinct purpose. It's always most effective when this purpose is self-directed, not imposed on you by external sources.

The Second Pearl:
A Very Distinct Purpose

Nick Yphantides, M.D.

I had the pleasure of meeting Dr. Nick Yphantides at a wellness conference in San Diego. Ken Blanchard was the keynote speaker and delivered an inspirational message that addressed all of the positive health and fitness changes he had made in the previous year.

After the conference, "Dr. Nick" told me that at one point he had weighed nearly 500 pounds. That was hard for me to imagine because in a business suit, he appeared to be of very normal, fit proportions. As he began to tell me his story, I recalled from earlier press releases that he was the physician who had lost 270 pounds in a year and had written a book entitled *My Big Fat Greek Diet* (2004). I told him about my project with Ken, and we immediately struck up a friendship. After reading his book, I interviewed him about his incredible journey.

I felt comfortable enough with Dr. Nick to ask him how it was that he became a 467-pound family physician.

He replied, "I was a board-certified medical hypocrite proclaiming to my patients every day, 'Do as I say, not as I do.' I did my best to fit my size into my reputation of being a 'big man with a huge heart,' as I was a physician to the poor and uninsured. I was viewed as a gentle giant—a medical teddy bear. I was living a life of profound hypocrisy in both my personal health and my public medical career.

There was a major disconnect between my words and my actions.

"My problem was that I was practicing what I call *food idolatry*. Food had become so much more than a source of nutrition for me—it was like my god. Food was where I turned to deal with my stress, loneliness, boredom, anxiety, and lack of intimacy. Food, of course, should not be Valium on a plate. Food is not your best friend. Food is not where you should turn to deal with uncertainty. Yet, sadly, food became all that and more for me. I used it as a crutch, as a soothing blanket, and as a means of numbing pain and escaping from reality. And yet I projected a happy, jolly man of healing whom many found quite appealing and desirable. Unfortunately, I was suffering as I imploded under the weight of my body and my daily hypocrisy.

"Over time, my weight had gradually crept upward in such a way that I didn't notice the magnitude of the problem. I knew I was large, but since the scale at home peaked out at 350 pounds, I assumed I weighed approximately that much. The only way I could accurately weigh myself was to place two scales side by side, put one foot on each, hold my breath, and add the two numbers together. The first time I did this, I was so shocked at the result of my calculations that I had to get on and off the scales several times to be sure it was accurate—467 pounds!

"I had a size 60 waist with a very limited wardrobe. I was a physician and a political leader who was forced to dress very informally. I was unable to fit into an airplane seat. I drove an oversized car out of necessity. I always hoped for the aisle seat at a ball game, movie, or play. I dreaded going to an unfamiliar restaurant, afraid I might not fit into a booth or a chair with arms. I was judged and assumed to be a slob or a lazy couch potato, and often ignored as unattractive and undesirable. I couldn't go to the beach, wear shorts, or be comfortable in many social situations. I could barely make it up one flight of steps without getting winded. I overcompensated with humor, publicly cracking jokes about myself. Such were my feelings and thoughts, and the facts of my life as a 467-pound, quarter-ton man.

"Then I was hit with a harsh reality. Only 31 years of age and still single, I had an unexpected bout with testicular cancer that finally forced me to deal with the consequences of my daily decisions. Although the cancer diagnosis was unrelated to my obesity problem, for the first time in my life I was compelled to face my own mortality head-on. As a result, I suddenly saw that my physical health was a God-given gift over which I had an obligation to demonstrate good stewardship. As I now look back on that dramatic time, I realize that cancer was a blessing that actually saved my life.

"Fortunately, I recovered from the cancer—but it dawned on me how ironic it was that I was still slowly killing myself with an avalanche of calories and lack of exercise. Although the cancer was not something I had direct control over, my weight problem and its associated risks of heart disease, diabetes, arthritis, and high blood pressure were things I could actually change. My cancer diagnosis became the catalyst for a new way of life."

I asked Dr. Nick for advice he would give to people who are extremely overweight and want to regain their health and fitness.

Dr. Nick said, "My bottom line is this: you have to change the way you *see* before you can change the way you *look*.

It's a play on words but it makes a key point. To change our weight, we have to change our life. To change our health, we have to change our routines. And change is hard—for many it may seem impossible. Start by spending a few minutes taking inventory. Is the pain of where you are now enough for you to tolerate the pain and discomfort of change? We all have to be motivated appropriately and meaningfully. If you are comfortable with where you are, it's very unlikely you're going to be willing to make meaningful changes. But if you're sick and tired of being sick and tired and are ready for a new way of life, embrace change.

"There is no 'one size fits all.' We all have different things to change. You say you don't have time? Make time. We all do for what is important. You say you can't afford to do it? Be honest! Can you afford *not* to do it? You say you feel as if getting healthy would be selfish? Get real! Being *unhealthy* is being selfish because we are depriving ourselves and those around us of what could be. And, to put it bluntly, some of us are facing premature death and will leave behind grieving children and grandchildren because we could not—or would not—change our ways. Being healthy is being loving. Give your spouse 20 pounds for her birthday! Give your grandkids 10 pounds each for the holidays! Embrace change and live life. I look back on my past routine and realize the life I was living was one of deprivation and frustration. Living healthy is so much more delicious and redemptive."

If you have an extreme overweight condition, I highly recommend you read Nick's book, *My Big Fat Greek Diet*. It is highly motivational and describes his story of losing weight and regaining health with a very compelling purpose.

Note from Tim: It should be noted that Dr. Nick lost nearly 300 pounds in less than a year on a low-calorie meal replacement diet. *Ken and I do not recommend this kind of diet unless you are under strict medical supervision.* Dr. Nick, a physician himself, was under the direct supervision of his brother, who is a board-certified family physician.

The Third Pearl: Sometimes Good Genetics Play a Role

Dorothy "Dodo" Cheney
International Tennis Hall of Fame Member

During the 20 years I owned my fitness business, I had the opportunity to work with many people well into their second half of life who had never worked out seriously before. It would always amaze me to see what good shape some of them could be in without having done regular exercise.

As the title of this section states, sometimes good genes do play a role. I recall hearing a number of times in the health and fitness industry that genetics can account for about 50 percent of a person's potential longevity. This means if someone has relatively poor genes (e.g., a family history of heart disease, cancer, diabetes, or other life-threatening disease) accounting for 50 percent of their longevity, and the other 50 percent is a matter of environmental situations and choices, that person will need to be diligent about health and fitness to have the best chance at a long life. On the other hand—even though we should all make healthy choices—if someone's ancestors lived long lives and few of the aforementioned health problems exist in the family history, that person may be able to focus more on getting the most out of life.

Dorothy "Dodo" Cheney is an example of the latter scenario. I was able to arrange an interview with her and was eager to hear about her secrets to a long and successful life.

In 2012 at age 97, Dodo Cheney finally had to quit playing tennis. After winning her 394th national tennis championship, she came to the unwelcome realization that her inability to balance was affecting her play. She reluctantly decided she needed to give up her favorite pastime before she had a bad fall.

Dodo came from a lineage of tennis stars. In 1905, her mother, May Sutton Bundy, was the first American woman to win Wimbledon, and she won it again in 1907. Dodo began playing tennis at age 8, won her first tournament at age 10, and became the first American to win the women's singles title at the Australian Open in 1938. She was inducted into the International Tennis Hall of Fame in 2004.

I asked her if she did a lot of conditioning work besides tennis. She answered, "No, but I played tennis every day and as many tournaments as I could handle."

She said she never let a minor injury get in the way and never made excuses. Dodo always loved people and loved to compete. She is obviously a D4—self-reliant achiever at tennis, but she told me she never would have been as good as she was without a great support system.

Dodo's daughter, Christie, summed up her mother's winning philosophies:

- Laugh a lot and have fun!
- Never make excuses.
- Always keep a competitive spirit.
- Have a strong support system.
- Keep stress to a minimum.
- Don't let your age become a limiting factor.
- As you age, practice mental gymnastics.

Since she no longer plays tennis, Dodo's new passion is besting everyone at Scrabble. During our interview, I noticed that her mind is unquestionably razor sharp. At 97, she still lives in her own house and loves gardening.

As I stood up to leave, Dodo said with a twinkle in her eye, "Hey, Tim, want to play a little tennis before you go?"

After first thinking about her decision to retire from the game, and then about the pounding my ego would take when she crushed me on the court—as she surely would—I replied with a smile, "No, thanks!"

The Fourth Pearl: Making the Ultimate Commitment

Dr. Lee Rice
Ken's Personal Physician

I interviewed Dr. Lee Rice, Ken's personal physician, about Ken's fitness journey. I began by asking him for his observations of Ken's commitment to fitness over the years.

He replied, "Ken has made numerous attempts at becoming fit over the past 30 years, but he has never lasted more than a couple of months. What's different this time? In all probability, a number of things. You, Tim, have been a very influential coach and source of hope and inspiration for him. Monitoring his progress and holding him accountable have been powerfully effective tools. The fact that he likes and trusts you is also very important.

"Ken is also tired of losing this battle and wants to succeed. He's older now and understands that the state of his health and fitness has become progressively influential in determining how long he will live and how functional he will be. Ken's orthopedic surgeon insisted that Ken lose weight before his joint replacements, so that was incentivizing. Since those procedures, it has been easier for Ken to move and exercise due to a more normal posture and gait, so that has helped significantly.

"Ken has had tons of support from family, friends, and his men's group—a committed group of men who meet monthly to help each other learn and grow and who would do anything to help Ken reach his full life's potential. His faith in God has been unwavering, and I think he wants to practice what he preaches in terms of honoring the gift of his life by returning his best on behalf of the world. Now he wants more and has hope and belief that he can truly be successful. Hope and expectation are extremely important.

"He joined Weight Watchers, which I believe has contributed a lot. His son Scott was instrumental by sharing his 'tough love' truth with his father. I think that was very impacting and made Ken face reality. He has finally accepted the truth that he can't be successful for a lifetime unless he trusts the process, gets his own ego out of the way, surrenders to the truth, accepts help from others, and commits to a consistent nutritional, exercise, and behavioral program that mirrors his spiritual belief system."

Next, I pointed out to Dr. Rice how Ken, a successful author and speaker, obviously has the means to surround himself with a community of health and fitness experts. I asked him what he has found to be the key components for the average person to achieve an optimal level of fitness. Here is his list:

- A clear understanding of your own values and priorities in life
- A willingness to align your personal behaviors with your values and priorities
- Absolute commitment and dedication to success, as opposed to being "interested" in success
- A coach, mentor, accountability buddy, or team
- A commitment to rigorous honesty
- Clear, measurable, and attainable goal setting

- Attaching your fitness goals to a higher life purpose than just getting fit or losing weight—for example, envisioning someday walking your daughter down the aisle as opposed to just wanting to lose 10 pounds
- A system of monitoring, accountability, and clarity on key indicators of success
- Constant reassessment and redirection
- Celebrating small successes along the way
- An ability to live "in the now"
- Eliminating negative self-talk
- Constantly reframing your personal experience to reflect positive self-worth, gratitude, hope, and love
- Never giving up

Dr. Rice ended by saying, "We are all addicted to the habits we practice. In order to change these ingrained habits, we first must give ourselves permission to change. Then we must believe—truly believe—that we are capable of much more. Peter Drucker, the corporate philosopher, said that for true transformational change, we need to have a complete break from the past. Most people want to gradually lean into change so that it doesn't make them or others too uncomfortable. This rarely works in the long run. I like to encourage people to dream big, envision the meaning of success in their effort, and wholeheartedly go for it. Announce the goal, put a stake in the ground, and be committed. Remove the obstacles that have been the seeds to past failures. Pave the way for success, and don't be afraid to make the critical choices and changes that will ensure success. Let go of fear. Expect problems and don't become paralyzed by temporary setbacks or failures. Learn from past mistakes and use them as a means to learn and grow. Be grateful for the lessons, enjoy the path, and embrace love."

RESOURCES II
Understanding Exercise and Fitness: Tim's Toolbox

This appendix gives you a more in-depth overview of the components of fitness that I've shared throughout this book. Even if you already have a good knowledge of fitness, you may want to review this section anyway.

—Tim Kearin

A Guide to the
Components of Fitness

Because the qualifications to be a fitness trainer do not require a license, there are many different approaches and philosophies to fitness. Just because some people look lean and muscular doesn't necessarily mean they know what they are doing. The industry has numerous trainer certification courses where the basics of physiology and anatomy are taught along with safety concerns and CPR. Most universities and colleges offer bachelor's, master's and even Ph.D. degrees in many sports science areas, including kinesiology, exercise physiology, biomechanics, and several other exercise disciplines. When seeking out a trainer, it is always a good idea to check the résumé, which should include at least a bachelor's degree and several years of experience working with individuals in your age group. It is also a good idea to check a reference or two.

My philosophy is based on formal education, personal experience, and many years as a competitor, strength coach, clinic director, and business owner. My core discipline was developed at the United States Military Academy. I arrived there at the tail end of a comprehensive strength training study cosponsored by Nautilus. All components of strength training were tested: men versus women, high reps versus low reps, speed of repetitions, time between sets, specific exercises, recovery time, and several other parameters. At the academy, this evolved into seven strength training variables. Most of the individuals involved in the study were young, healthy, and highly motivated. Using these variables certainly produced results, but I have found when training myself and numerous clients over the years that adaptations have to be made as you get older.

How the Body Metabolizes Energy

Before we get into the mechanics of a program, it is important to understand how our body metabolizes energy. At rest, our heart beats at the rate of approximately 70 beats per minute (70 bpm). Our resting metabolism represents the amount of energy required to maintain bodily functions and keep our core temperature at about 98.6 degrees. While sleeping or at rest, our heart rate is 60 to 70 bpm, and we are burning about one calorie per minute. This is the basis for our basic metabolic rate (BMR). Males burn calories at a slightly higher rate than females, mostly because they have a greater muscle mass. Most males would have a BMR of about 1,400 calories per day, and most females would have a BMR of about 1,200 calories. These numbers are important when we discuss weight loss later.

In terms of fuel, our body has three primary energy sources: (1) fat—an almost endless supply stored mainly in fatty banks all around the body; (2) glucose—a much lesser supply stored in the muscles and liver; and (3) ATP (adenosine triphosphate)—a very limited supply stored in the muscle cells. For fat and glucose, combustion (muscle contraction) occurs when oxygen combines with the fuel source. The by-product (burned fuel) becomes carbon dioxide and is carried away in the bloodstream. The by-product of ATP is lactic acid (incomplete sugar burn), which blocks the muscles' ability to contract. Fat is the preferred energy source when the body is at rest and continues until we are working at about 65 percent of our predicted maximum heart rate.

For simple calculations of your predicted maximum heart rate, take the number 220—which is said to be our maximum heart rate at birth—and subtract your age. For example, a 50-year-old would subtract 50 from 220 and have a predicted maximum heart rate of 170 bpm. When we exercise hard enough to exceed 65 percent—111 bpm for our 50-year-old—our body can no longer provide enough fat for combustion so the body calls for glucose. From 65 percent to approximately 85 percent—111 to 144 bpm for our 50-year-old—our body will use glucose as the energy source. Beyond 85 percent—145 bpm for our 50-year-old—our body shifts to ATP. These all have considerable training implications.

The First Component of Fitness: Aerobic Exercise

Aerobic exercise is necessary for the health of the heart, lungs, and circulation. And as many people know, it's the best way to burn stored body fat.

Because I am an exercise fanatic, I always look for a gym right away when I travel. Being a gym owner, I always like to go in with a guest pass, with no one knowing who I am, and enjoy watching how people work out. One of the things I frequently observe is seeing an apparently unconditioned individual working on a Stairmaster machine going on level 10, holding on for dear life, sweating like crazy, breathing excessively, and running totally out of gas in about 10 minutes. If you have ever been in a large gym I'm sure you have observed this as well. Upon completion, the person can hardly stand up and is gasping for air, announcing what a great workout it was. The reality is that this person just wasted 15 minutes and put him- or herself at risk.

Let's examine this scenario: By going from rest (70 bpm) to 90 percent almost immediately, people who exercise in this way bypass the ability to operate aerobically and use fat as a fuel source. Instead, they require the body to use ATP (stored muscle energy) and operate anaerobically. Because ATP is in short supply and they are generating lactic acid, they can only keep this up for a very short period. Now they drop the workload back because they have to. At best, they are burning glucose for fuel and never tap into their fat sources. They walk around feeling light-headed as the body attempts to pay back oxygen debt and dissipate lactic acid. They usually feel too bad to continue the workout. This feeling does not motivate them to come back. In addition, because they have depleted blood glucose, they crave sugar for replenishment—which ultimately gets converted to body fat.

Burning fat. Let's look at a more practical approach: Most of us have enough fat stored to walk around the world without replenishment. We store enough glucose to last about two hours before depletion and enough ATP to last less than a minute. Given that most of us desire to lose body fat, doesn't it make more sense to do a program that will burn fat as the primary fuel? Let's take a look at how we would do that.

If you are just starting out—having received a clearance from your physician—a simple walk around the block should suffice, particularly if you are overweight and out of shape.

Your objective should be to walk slowly on a flat surface as long as you can go without breathing too hard. If you cannot carry on a normal conversation without gasping for air between words, you are walking too fast.

Once you can do this for 15 minutes, you should start monitoring your pulse. Before you walk, figure out your target range. As stated earlier, take the number 220 and subtract your age, then multiply it by 60 percent. When you have walked for five minutes, stop and take your pulse. The easiest way to do this is to stop and place your index finger and middle finger next to your Adam's apple and when you feel a pulse, count for 15 seconds on your watch and multiply that number by four.

EXAMPLE: A 50-year-old person

$220 - 50 = 170 \times 60\% = 102$ bpm. A good starting point!

Another alternative is to buy a pulse monitor. It consists of a rubber strip that straps around your chest with a telemetry device on the front that will send the signal to a wrist monitor. These devices cost from $50 to $75 and provide a very easy and accurate means of monitoring your pulse rate. Once you are able to calculate your heart rate, you should do an aerobic exercise a minimum of three times per week for 20 minutes. There is almost no such thing as too much. As you become better conditioned, a good goal would be to do 30 to 60 minutes three times per week on alternate days. Eventually, if you have the time, do an aerobic activity six days per week.

Aerobic activity: Walking. One of the best aerobic activities is something we do every day just to get around—

walking. At rest, our heart beats approximately 70 times per minute and we are burning 1 calorie of fat. If we never moved our bodies, we would burn about 1,440 calories per day. If we increase our walking speed, our heart rate will increase to meet the new demand for fuel. If our heart rate increases to 60 percent of our predicted maximum heart rate, our calorie burn increases to 3 to 5 calories per minute, and we are still using fat as the primary fuel source. If we increase our walking workload enough to get our heart rate to 80 percent, we are now burning 7 to 10 calories per minute. We are still burning some fat but now need more carbohydrate to help because the exercise intensity has increased. The reason for the range on the calorie burn is that we burn more calories when we are better conditioned.

As mentioned earlier in the book, a great tool to help you get and stay motivated is a pedometer. You clip it on your belt or waistband, and it counts the number of steps you take in a day. A good goal to shoot for is 10,000 steps per day. That sounds impossible, but I have tried it and with a normal day, including 40 minutes of exercise, I easily exceed this mark. Once you have achieved that goal, shoot for 70,000 per week. You will be amazed at how this practice will contribute to fat loss.

If you choose walking for the aerobic component, a walking partner can really help with camaraderie. The days in between you could do strength training exercises. This is where a fitness trainer can help establish your recommended program.

Aerobic activity: Running. When I was younger, I hated aerobic exercise. I always thought of aerobic activity as running, which didn't seem to complement the weight lifting that

I did. It wasn't until I arrived at West Point that I really appreciated the importance of endurance conditioning. Everyone ran at West Point. In fact, as an army officer you were tested every year on your ability to do the two-mile run.

Running really wasn't my thing, but as I got into my 30s, I did begin to appreciate the benefits. More than anything I liked the way it made me feel and the way it kept my body lean. Now in my early 60s, aerobic activity has become a priority. My primary motivation is keeping my heart healthy. While I was at West Point, my father died of a massive heart attack at age 61. His history suggested that he did exercise a little from my urging but was 30 pounds overweight and had high blood pressure, high cholesterol, and high stress. His passing became my motivation to do at least 30 minutes of aerobic exercise five to six days per week. I've been doing that for the past 30 years, and my blood pressure and cholesterol have remained low as a result. I still don't like aerobic exercise but love the benefits and will continue it for as long as I'm physically capable.

One thing that has really helped me is to get more creative. I gave up running following back surgery at age 49. If I'm in a gym, there's no way I can stay on a treadmill and watch the seconds tick away. To me that is like watching grass grow. What I usually do is get on the exercise bike for 10 minutes, move to the elliptical cross-trainer for 10 minutes, and then go to the treadmill and walk on a grade for the final 10 minutes. With that routine, the boredom factor is gone and time moves rather quickly. As long as I don't stop between strength training exercises and keep my heart rate at target, I'm actually getting more benefit—because I'm doing what is called *cross training*. The body is a very efficient machine. If you always do the same routine, your body will try to conserve and will actually use less energy.

I like to mix my gym workouts with long hikes on the weekend. This is something my wife and I do together. We live in hilly terrain in San Diego and will sometimes hike for as long as two hours. The advantage of walking or hiking outside is the change of scenery and the fresh air.

Other aerobic activities. Cycling, swimming, singles tennis, rollerblading, cross-country skiing, spinning, and aerobic dancing are also great aerobic activities. My wife Sharon is a dancer and has been teaching aerobic dance classes for years. The classes are great because they build camaraderie and accountability and they are fun. The objective is to keep the heart rate at a steady 60 to 70 percent range for 20 minutes to an hour. Along with doing mixed activities, it is also beneficial to push to 70 to 80 percent once in a while.

The Second Component of Fitness: Strength Training

To keep muscles from atrophy (shrinking in size) and to prevent bone loss as you age, it's important to add strength training to your fitness program. In the 1970s, Nautilus Corporation did an extensive strength training research study at West Point using the cadets as subjects, which led to the development of what is called the Seven Strength Training Variables. After 35 years, I still follow these principles. Here is a brief description:

Sets. This refers to the total number of repetitions performed in a given exercise. The number of sets varies with the type of equipment used. If fatigue is achieved through the entire range of motion, such as with a cam-accommodated machine, then only one set is necessary. If a barbell or dumbbell is used, additional sets may be required as only the weakest portion in the range of motion reaches fatigue in the first set.

Reps. This is the number of times you move the resistance through the full range of motion. There are two parts of the repetition. The first part of the movement involves a shortening contraction of the muscle and is called a *concentric* contraction. The second part, where the muscle lengthens while lowering the resistance, is called the *eccentric* phase. Here are some recommended reps for general training purposes:

Age 20 to 40: 8 to 12 reps
Age 41 to 60: 12 to 15 reps
Age 60 and above: 15 to 20 reps

Even though muscle tissue continues to regenerate, we become weaker because of inactivity and bone and cartilage loss. Therefore, it is best to achieve fatigue at a higher number of reps, which puts less stress on the joint.

Weight. This refers to the amount of resistance. It should be enough to cause muscle fatigue within the repetition range mentioned. When you can do the highest number in the rep range, you should increase the resistance by about 10 percent. If done properly, this approach should reduce the set to the bottom on the repetition range. As we continue to increase, we call this *progressive resistance training.*

Speed of reps. Numerous theories describe how fast a repetition should be performed. The extremes go from moving the weight as fast as you can, such as the "power clean" in weight lifting, to "superslow" training where each rep can take 45 seconds to complete. The Nautilus study at West Point suggested two seconds for the lifting phase, a pause at the extreme point, and four seconds for the lowering phase. It's my opinion that you should move the weight at a speed where momentum does not become involved.

Time between sets. If you are doing more than one set of the same exercise, you should allow at least two minutes for the lactic acid to circulate out of the muscle before repeating. If you are not repeating the same exercise or doing opposing exercises, no wait is necessary. A technique that is commonly practiced by weight lifters is called super-setting. This is where you immediately follow an exercise by doing the opposing movement exercise (e.g., a chest press and a seated row). Such a practice actually increases circulation to and from the opposing muscle group.

Recovery between workouts. When you fatigue muscles in the manner just described, you need to allow at least 48 hours for recovery. The muscle stress causes tiny tears in the fibers, and they rebuild stronger than before. Usually when people begin a program they will work out in this manner three times per week. After three months, twice per week is adequate for maintenance.

What exercises and what order of exercises. You need to work as many major muscle groups as possible. When practical, you should work the larger muscles and multiple joint exercises first. Then do the smaller muscles and isolation exercises next.

Circuit training. Being an older man, I regard this as my favorite way of training. It maximizes time and you kill two birds with one stone—probably not a good analogy in the health business! There are many ways to do circuit training. One way is to go to a class where you have a number of strength training stations set up with an aerobic station in between. The instructor blows a whistle at 60-second intervals, and you alternate a strength exercise with an aerobic exercise, thereby getting mutual benefits for the same time allotment.

My favorite way is to set the treadmill at a moderate level and every two minutes leave the treadmill to perform a strength exercise. This way, in 40 minutes I've completed 12 strength exercises and kept my heart rate in the target zone by doing aerobic exercise in between. This can create certain logistical problems in a gym because of other participants in the way, but if you have a more private situation, this is the best way to train. I will note that this technique is more advanced and should be set up by a trainer to ensure that it is the most efficient program and that you are physically capable.

The Third Component of Fitness: Flexibility

To keep limbs mobile and avoid injuries, it's important to maintain flexibility. A good flexibility program should include stretching the arms and shoulders, the lower back and trunk, and the legs. You should attempt to isolate each joint and move slowly until there is a slight burning or stretching feeling. Hold that position and breathe deeply and exhale for 15 seconds, then release for 15 seconds and repeat, attempting to go a little further the next time. It is a fact that warm muscles are more mobile than cold muscles, so it is always a good idea to do at least five minutes of light aerobic work first.

A question that frequently comes up is *Should I stretch before I work out?* Research has shown that static stretching before exercise is less efficient than after exercise. For this reason, I have always done stretching at the end of the workout. It is not only more productive, it also serves as a cool-down. This is another situation where your trainer can set up a good program for you.

A wonderful flexibility practice is yoga, which not only keeps the body limber but also improves balance, concentration, and serenity. Because of the many subtle elements of yoga, it's a difficult practice to learn on your own. A good yoga teacher is worth seeking out, and you might very well find some kindred spirits to become part of your fitness support group.

The Fourth Component of Fitness: Balance Training

One of the great perils of aging is falling, so balance is an essential component of being fit—especially as you get older.

A number of tests can measure your ability to balance, but the most common test is one you can do on your own at home. Have someone stand by you as a spotter and see how long you can balance standing on one foot only. Try this initially with your eyes open while standing next to a counter or anything stable above hip level to grab onto. Look straight ahead and count the number of seconds you can balance without needing help. Try standing on the dominant leg first, and then the nondominant leg. Most people can balance longer on the dominant leg; however, I've noticed how golfers usually balance longer on the leg that is opposite of the side they swing from. For example, a right-handed golfer would balance longer on the left leg. I suspect this is the result of always placing more weight on the opposite leg.

There are a number of other tests conducted by personal trainers and physical therapists, but I think standing on one leg is a good practical indicator that you can do by yourself. If you can't balance at all without holding on to something, or if you can balance for only a few seconds, you definitely need work. Strength training exercises that strengthen the buttocks, hip flexors, hip abductors and adductors, quadriceps, hamstrings, and calves will definitely help. However, if you can't balance for at least 30 seconds on each leg, you should be doing supplemental balance exercises daily if possible. The best training involves fall-risk exercises but should only be done with a trainer. Here are some exercises you can do on your own:

Single-leg stand. Stand with feet shoulder width apart, arms out to the sides and raise one leg off the ground. While using your arms as counterbalances, attempt to stand for as long as you can while looking straight ahead. Do the weaker side first and switch back and forth two to three times. Once you can stand for 30 seconds, try closing your eyes.

Single-leg stand with movement. Same as the single-leg stand, only move opposite leg out to the side then move the arms slowly around. Once you have mastered this, pick up a weighted object like a medicine ball and move it to front, sides, and then slowly overhead while balancing on one foot.

Walking a line. Locate or place a straight line with masking tape on the floor and walk on top of the line, placing one foot directly in front of the other. After walking 10 feet, do the same thing walking backward.

Golfers. One of the reasons golfers have difficulty hitting the ball as they get older is because their balance becomes worse. To correct this condition, I have subjects stand on one foot, hold a golf club as they would when addressing the ball, and raise one foot off the ground. When they have achieved balance, I have them gently swing the golf club back and forth. Once they can do this from either foot, their ability to address the ball and hit it squarely dramatically improves.

Several other more advanced balance exercises, such as balancing on a BOSU ball, are available, but they involve considerable fall risk and should be done with a trainer.

The Fifth Component of Fitness: Nutrition and Weight Control

No matter how much you exercise, unless you focus attention on nutrition and weight control, you'll never attain optimum health.

Nutrition

Protein. Proteins are necessary for the repair of damaged muscle and bone tissue. The amount required for the average person who doesn't exercise is about 0.8 grams of protein per kilogram of body weight. This would suggest that a 150-pound person would require about 50 grams per day. If that same 150-pound person were doing serious strength training, which causes micro tears to the muscle tissues, they would require about 1.5 grams of protein per kilogram of body weight or 100 grams. Protein provides the amino acids, which are the building blocks of damaged tissues. The body does not really have a storage capacity for additional protein, so the excess is excreted from the body. Foods that are a good source of protein are lean meats, poultry, fish, unprocessed cheese, nonfat milk, nuts, and soy beans. If you eat properly, protein supplements are generally unnecessary. It is also a good idea to eat protein with every meal.

Carbohydrates. Carbohydrates are highly misunderstood. I believe the general feeling is that you should always be on low carbs if you are trying to lose weight. Carbs are necessary for maintaining blood glucose and glycogen storage. However, it is important to understand that there are good carbs and bad carbs. The bad carbs are the starches and refined sugars—just about everything that is white. Starches are generally loaded with calories, have very little nutritional value, and do little to satisfy your hunger. Because of the instant release of insulin, digestion becomes difficult. The body does need sugar, but the best sources are found directly in nature. Vegetables, fruits, and whole-grain products are good sources. These have to be broken down in the body's digestive tract and are processed into glucose in a slow, controlled manner. Our 150-pound inactive person would need about 150 to 200 grams of carbohydrate for brain and muscle function and the same-sized athlete might need 300 to 400 grams of carbohydrate. Carbs also should be ingested with every meal or between meals.

Fats. Just like carbohydrates, there are good fats (unsaturated) and there are bad fats (saturated). Your body needs some saturated fat, but it should only account for about one-third of your fat intake. Fat has many functions: it is our primary source of energy while functioning at normal levels of activity; it provides vitamins A, D, E, and K; it is responsible for the development of cell structure, and it provides us with insulation (usually too much). There is no minimum or maximum amount published, but fat generally should constitute about 30 percent of our diet. Good sources of unsaturated fats come from vegetable oils, olive oils, canola oils, nuts, and fatty fishes like salmon and sardines.

Water. We generally don't think of water as a nutritional item, but without it we would cease to exist. The adult body is approximately 70 percent water—of which about 80 percent is stored in muscle and 20 percent in fat. It is recommended that we drink eight glasses of water, or approximately one-half of our body weight number in ounces, per day. This is difficult and takes a conscious effort for most people, but proper hydration is necessary for body functions. Our electrolyte balance is greatly affected by our hydration level. If our electrolytes are too low, we experience muscle cramping and other systemic dysfunctions. You will frequently observe this early in the football season when top athletes have to leave the game because of muscle cramping. This is caused by massive sweating and improper hydration. That is why you will frequently see them drinking sports drinks that are loaded with electrolyte replacement. When doing aerobic exercise, it is important to drink small amounts of water frequently during the workout. It is best to drink cool water as it is more easily absorbed than ice water.

Supplements

Vitamins. Most foods that we eat these days are fortified with vitamins. A nutritionally sound diet will generally provide the RDA requirement for vitamins. If in doubt, a good multivitamin will ensure that all bases are covered.

Glucosamine and Chondroitin. These are said to enhance joint health in the aging population. I once heard an orthopedic surgeon say that when he does joint surgery, he can tell who is taking it. There are no known side effects that I have heard of. My experience is that most middle-aged and older people are taking it in some form.

Deer Antler Extract. This is a whole food product that is made up of ground up deer antlers after they have been shed. It is helpful with the regeneration of cartilage. It has glucosamine/chondroitin, hyaluronic acid, collagen, prostaglandins, and other growth factors. The Chinese have been using it effectively for thousands of years.

Weight Control

Weight Control by Exercise Alone. If you read the section on metabolism, you learned that weight control is the result of calories in versus calories out. The formula works like this: one pound of fat is equal to 3,500 calories. If you are consuming 3,000 calories per day and your output is equal to 2,500, you have a surplus of 500, which suggests that you will gain 1 pound of fat every 7 days, or 4 pounds per month. Let's assume that we are maintaining weight and would like to lose 10 pounds. Here is how we would accomplish that with exercise alone:

We are burning 1,400 calories with our basic metabolic rate (BMR). Let's say we burn another 1,600 doing our normal daily activities. Our body weight is constant, suggesting that we are expending 3,000 calories per day. If we begin to exercise for 45 minutes per day, with enough intensity to burn 5 to 6 calories per minute (250), then we will create a deficit of 250 per day, or 3,500 calories every 2 weeks. That equals 2 pounds per month and 25 pounds in 1 year. A slow process, but it works.

Weight Control by Diet Alone. Whenever we go on a diet, it is generally for the purpose of losing weight. This is accomplished by taking in fewer calories than we burn. Using the same scenario as above and reducing our intake by 500 calories, with everything else being the same, we will lose one pound per week. The key to this scenario is the phrase "everything else being the same." This is why diet plans that provide packaged foods are effective—they have a precise calorie count. When weight is lost this fast without exercise, the result is often that pear-shaped look. The downside of packaged foods is that you seldom learn how to cut your own calories and often all weight is gained back as soon as the diet is over.

Many people will skip meals such as breakfast, thinking they are limiting calories. This is a form of fasting, which is ineffective and counterproductive. The body senses it isn't getting enough food, so it goes into a conservation mode and the metabolism slows down. When the next large meal is consumed, the body wants to convert it to fat and store it, because it doesn't know when the next meal is coming. Dieting without exercise will result in weight loss, but it seldom lasts.

Weight Control by Diet and Exercise. This is the best and by far the most accepted method for losing weight. If you decrease your caloric intake by 500 calories per day and do 45 minutes per day of aerobic exercise, the result will be six pounds lost per month. If strength training is done two to three times per week in addition to the aerobic work, you are developing more calorie burners as well as developing the appropriate shape.

The most effective way to diet is to become nutritionally smart and learn the basics of your body's requirements. If you eat smaller, more frequent meals, your body senses it is getting too much food and wants to burn it off. This is not always the most convenient way to eat, but is the accepted practice of almost all diet plans. Another trick is to always leave something on your plate. An obvious and logical method is to give up desserts. A basic knowledge of nutrition, when combined with exercise, will help shape you and keep the weight off.

The Sixth Component of Fitness: Rest and Sleep

Sleep plays an important role in health and fitness. Ken's friend, Dr. James B. Maas, is an expert on sleep. A former professor and past chairman of the psychology department at Cornell, Maas is coauthor of the book *Sleep for Success!* (2011), which became an instant classic on the topic of sleep. His latest book is *Sleep to Win! Secrets to Unlocking Your Athletic Excellence in Every Sport* (2013).

Maas states that in a typical eight-hour night, if you sleep well, you'll experience four or five 90-minute sleep cycles before waking up for the day:

Waking Stage: Your body prepares for sleep. You're awake in this stage but very relaxed. Your eyes can be open or closed.

Sleep Stage 1: Drowsiness. At this stage—lasting anywhere from 10 seconds to 10 minutes—you transition from being awake to falling asleep. Your breathing becomes shallow and irregular. "People often say they are half asleep in this stage," says Maas. "You respond fairly quickly to disturbances, since you're still aware of your surroundings."

Sleep Stage 2: Light Sleep. During this stage, your eye movements come to a halt, your blood pressure drops, and your muscles relax more. "This is the actual beginning of sleep, because at this point you're no longer aware of your environment," says Maas.

Sleep Stages 3 and 4: Deep Sleep. In these two consecutive stages (stage 4 is slightly deeper), your body regenerates, repairs tissues, and develops bone and muscle. Deep sleep also gives your immune system a boost and restores the energy you've lost during the day. You'll be in deep sleep for 40 to 60 minutes. "If you are woken up in the middle of either of these stages, it'll take you about 20 seconds to realize where you are and what's happened," says Maas.

Sleep Stage 5: Rapid Eye Movement (REM) Sleep. The first REM period is short, lasting about nine minutes. But as the night goes on, each successive REM period doubles in length. Your eyes will move rapidly in different directions and while your brain is shut off from the outside world, it's still working at preserving memory. You're also dreaming, and if you awaken you'll remember your dream vividly. In fact, many people will wake up during or just after REM sleep, either to roll over or to get up and start their day.

Are you sleep deprived? Depriving the brain of sleep "makes you clumsy, stupid, and unhealthy," according to Maas. "Most adults are moderately to severely sleep deprived, and this affects their productivity, their work, and their relationships. If we treated machines like we treat the human body, we would be accused of reckless endangerment. We've become walking zombies—stressed and stretched to our limits. We can't fall asleep, we can't maintain sleep, we wake up too early, or some combination of all three. All of this has profound effects on our productivity and general well-being."

How do you know if you're sleep deprived? Maas suggests you consider your answers to these questions:

- Are you drowsy during the day?
- Does a warm room, boring meeting, heavy meal, or low dose of alcohol make you drowsy?
- Do you fall asleep within five minutes of hitting the pillow?
- Do you need an alarm clock to wake up?
- Do you often hit the snooze bar?
- Do you sleep extra hours on the weekend?

If you answered yes to two or more of those questions, you should consider yourself pathologically sleep deprived—and you should do something about it.

What's so bad about being sleep deprived, you ask? "There are serious, deleterious health consequences," warns Maas. "You're at a higher risk for hypertension—that's heart attacks and strokes—type 2 diabetes, irritability, anxiety, depression, cancer, and obesity. Your reaction time is slower. You lose your sense of humor and your perspective. You have significantly lowered cognitive performance which can cause you to make stupid, poor decisions."

What's the solution? Maas suggests the following:

- Determine your sleep requirement and meet it every night. For most of us, that's getting one more hour of sleep than we are getting now.
- Establish a regular sleep/wake cycle. Go to bed and get up at the same time every day, including weekends.
- Get one long block of continuous sleep. Make sure your bedroom is quiet, dark, and cool. Avoid any caffeine after 2:00 in the afternoon and alcohol within three hours of bedtime.
- Get plenty of exercise.
- Reduce stress in your life as much as possible.

- Avoid the use of electronics within an hour of bed-time. Computers, tablets, and e-readers emanate "blue light" that can block the secretion of melatonin in your brain, thereby delaying sleep onset when you finally turn off the lights.
- If you can't get enough sleep at night, instead of drinking caffeinated beverages, power-nap for 15 minutes during the typical midday dip in your alertness.

Most people are aware of the importance of nutrition and exercise to overall good health. It's time everyone woke up to the truth about the importance of sleep. Sweet dreams!

It is very important to have a complete program that includes aerobic exercise, strength training, flexibility, balance training, nutrition/weight control, and rest/sleep. Some individuals might need emphasis in certain areas, but as with Ken, a balanced program should include each of the items detailed in this section.

Working Out While Traveling

As we have mentioned, one of the great challenges for Ken and me was the fact that he was constantly traveling. In fact, it's probably fair to say that during the yearlong project, Ken was away from home approximately 30 percent of the time. Obviously, if we dropped the program while he was away, we would not have had anywhere near the success we did.

In Ken's case, keeping with the program while traveling was best accomplished by having him work with a trainer when possible for program adherence and accountability. Ken doesn't lack self-discipline; but as you learned from his Situational Leadership® II model, he does better when someone works with him. This presented a challenge for me because all trainers have their own philosophy and like to sell their own ideas. I didn't have a problem when it was just a few sessions, but in the cases where I was gone for three weeks and when Ken was gone for two months, I felt it was important that the trainers follow my program carefully. More than anything, I wanted to be sure they knew Ken's capabilities and limitations. In each case, I had full cooperation.

If you will be away from home more than a few days, keep your exercise and health considerations a priority. That doesn't mean you shouldn't have a good time, but try to keep moderation in mind. An onsite trainer who is familiar with the equipment can be useful; but if you don't want to spend money on a trainer, most large hotels either have an onsite gym or are affiliated with one. Aerobic work is pretty easy to do because a treadmill is a treadmill and a bike is a bike. Strength training equipment can be a little more difficult because there are many different equipment manufacturers and all different types of equipment. Stay within your normal repetition range, and do at least the multiple joint exercises such as chest press, row or lat pull-down, and leg press. Even two workouts per week will be enough to maintain.

Common Training Injuries

Many training injuries are the result of strains to soft tissue (i.e., tendons, ligaments, and muscles). Tendons attach muscles to bones, muscles move joints, and ligaments attach bones to bones. It is important that you learn to recognize these types of injuries when they occur.

When an injury occurs, chemicals are released into the bloodstream, starting a process called inflammation.

Vessels dilate and blood carries nutrients to the injury site. This process is followed by the arrival of white blood cells, which carry away damaged cells so the tissue can begin to scar. Scar tissue is the way soft tissue heals. It is important to understand this, because if you leave the injury alone without consideration of the rehab process, scar tissue can impede the eventual movement of the joint. This is why, if you are in doubt about an injury, it is important to seek medical advice from your doctor.

If you are certain that an injury is minor, follow the acronym RICE:

Rest: *Allow the injury time to recover without straining it again.* In most cases this involves active rest, which means keeping the parts moving gently so scar tissue doesn't lock it in place.

Ice: *Ice should become the best friend of anyone who is training.* It not only inhibits swelling but also promotes deep vessel circulation. Never apply heat to an injury during the first 72 hours, as this promotes swelling and impedes the healing process. As soon as possible, apply an ice pack to the injury site and leave it there for 20 minutes. Do not exceed 20 minutes unless advised by your physician. Allow at least a 30-minute interval and repeat several times per day.

Compression: *Compression is accomplished with something equivalent to an elastic bandage wrap.* This will help prevent and reduce swelling. Always start the wrap at the distal point (far end). The wrap should be snug, but not too tight. You want to restrict the surface flow but still allow for deep circulation.

Elevation: *Elevate the injury site above heart level if possible.* This will help prevent swelling and pooling of fluids at or below the injury.

The most common training injuries for adults as we mature are what we call overuse injuries. The body doesn't recover as quickly as it once did, so even standard workouts can be too intense without adequate recovery time. This frequently results in muscle strains and tendinitis. Muscle strains occur when we do not warm up properly and when we place too much load on the muscle. When this occurs frequently, the tendons become inflamed, resulting in tendinitis. Information on how to prevent this from happening is presented in the "Strength Training" section.

Shin splints. Shin splints frequently occur when an individual begins a walking or running program. It usually begins with soreness along the front of the shin bone. If it becomes chronic, even slow walking is uncomfortable. A frequent cause is from a muscle imbalance between the calf muscles on the back and the tibialis muscles on the front.

Tennis elbow. This injury refers to just about any pain on or around the elbow. If you play golf, it is called golfer's elbow. In any case, it is a painful occurrence and affects tasks as simple as raising a cup of coffee. This, again, is frequently the result of a muscle imbalance.

Low-back pain. I could write an entire book on this subject. Usually at age 50 and over, this condition is brought on by degenerative joint disease, or osteoarthritis. I've been dealing with this issue personally for the past 20 years. I had corrective surgery in 1995; and while the surgery was a success, I was left with considerable arthritis. This would be classified as a wear-and-tear condition that generates inflammation and discomfort. Many people with this condition regularly take ibuprofen, a nonsteroidal anti-inflammatory drug, and others take glucosamine/chondroitin. I personally take deer antler extract and have had great success with it.

Muscle strain. This usually occurs when a load greater than the muscle is accustomed to causes a tear in the fibers. This is what Ken Blanchard experienced while playing golf, as we wrote about earlier. He hit the ground while swinging his driver, and the force caused a rupture in the muscle belly of his left arm. It resulted in a lot of pain and discoloration, but fortunately the MRI revealed that it was not a complete rupture. A complete rupture usually requires surgical correction. I know about this personally, having ruptured the distal end of both bicep tendons. In Ken's case, we treated the injury with ice for several days, integrating mild range-of-motion exercise and friction massage. We continued to work all other body parts not involving the bicep and did progressive rehab on the injured arm. In six weeks, Ken was back where he was before the injury—with no lasting effects.

Joint replacements. Obviously this is not an injury, but workouts during the recovery period will need to be modified just as if you were recovering from an injury. The most common joint replacements occur in the knees, hips, and shoulders. Following a total joint replacement, your workouts will require some modification, but you generally can do the same things you did before. Ken has had both hips replaced, and I have had a total shoulder joint replacement, and we both do complete body workouts. This is another situation where a consultation with a good trainer can help. In many cases, the motivation for joint replacement is simply to improve the quality of life.

Because of the improvement in Ken's level of fitness during this journey, he has managed to avoid the total knee replacement surgery he had been warned may be necessary. I know that was an important motivator for him.

Because many older adults want to continue to live independently, do what they enjoy, and live active lives, the number of hip and knee replacements has more than doubled in the last 15 years. The big questions are often: When should I do it? Do I carve six months out of my life now, or do I put it off with the risk that the procedure and recovery may be more difficult later? Be sure you talk over your specific circumstances and options with your physician so you can make a well-thought-out decision.

RESOURCES III
Developing Your Own
Fitness Program

Here are some helpful reminders to get you started and a tool you can use to measure your progress in each of the six fitness areas we have discussed.

Before beginning your fitness journey, we suggest you review Tim's section starting on page 63 entitled "Selecting the Right Program for You" to brush up on the elements you'll need to have in place when you start your program. Once you've accomplished the first four elements (having a compelling purpose, getting a medical checkup, becoming educated about fitness, and setting up your support system), you'll see that the final element you need to put in place is learning about and applying Situational Leadership® II, which is covered in detail in Ken's section that starts on page 27.

The first step in applying SLII® is to set SMART goals for yourself—specific, motivating, attainable, relevant, and trackable—so you know what you want to accomplish and when. (To reacquaint yourself, see page 29.)

The next step is to diagnose your present **development level** in each of the six areas of fitness by checking the appropriate box in the table below. Respond openly and honestly.

D1—*Enthusiastic Beginner*: Low competence, high commitment

D2—*Disillusioned Learner*: Low to some competence, low commitment

D3—*Capable but Cautious Performer*: Moderate to high competence, variable commitment

D4—*Self-Reliant Achiever*: High competence, high commitment

Aerobic Exercise	D1 ❏	D2 ❏	D3 ❏	D4 ❏
Strength Training	D1 ❏	D2 ❏	D3 ❏	D4 ❏
Flexibility	D1 ❏	D2 ❏	D3 ❏	D4 ❏

Balance Training	D1 ❏	D2 ❏	D3 ❏	D4 ❏
Nutrition/Weight Control	D1 ❏	D2 ❏	D3 ❏	D4 ❏
Rest/Sleep	D1 ❏	D2 ❏	D3 ❏	D4 ❏

The final step in applying SLII® is to determine the matching **leadership style** (help) you'll need for each area by checking the appropriate box in the table below. Remember that a D1 development level generally needs an S1 leadership style; a D2 generally needs an S2, a D3 generally needs an S3, and a D4 generally needs an S4.

S1—*Directing*: Leader shows and tells specifically how, gives frequent feedback

S2—*Coaching*: Leader explains why, asks individual for suggestions and participation

S3—*Supporting*: Individual makes decisions with leader; leader encourages and supports

S4—*Delegating*: Individual makes decisions with little direction or support

Aerobic Exercise	S1 ❏	S2 ❏	S3 ❏	S4 ❏
Strength Training	S1 ❏	S2 ❏	S3 ❏	S4 ❏
Flexibility	S1 ❏	S2 ❏	S3 ❏	S4 ❏
Balance Training	S1 ❏	S2 ❏	S3 ❏	S4 ❏
Nutrition/Weight Control	S1 ❏	S2 ❏	S3 ❏	S4 ❏
Rest/Sleep	S1 ❏	S2 ❏	S3 ❏	S4 ❏

After you've completed this assessment, you will want to confer with your chosen partner in fitness—either a supportive, knowledgeable friend or a fitness professional—to be sure they understand the development level and leadership style concepts of SLII®. We suggest they read this book, or at least chapter 2, to solidify their understanding of the importance of SLII® to your fitness journey. Continue to use these tables as you progress in your development in each of these areas—and celebrate every time you reach a new level!

We hope you are ready to begin your fitness journey with a strong feeling of commitment and determination, and we wish you success. It's *your* time to become fit at last—and to look and feel better, once and for all!

Acknowledgments

Ken Blanchard

As you can imagine, since it took a community to help me succeed in my fitness journey, I have a lot of people to acknowledge.

First of all, my coauthor and fitness partner, Tim. Without your support, this journey never would have happened. My family—Margie, son Scott, his wife Madeleine, daughter Debbie, and my grandkids Alec, Kyle, Kurtis, Atticus, and Hannah, and, of course, the famous Joy—you were key motivators for my journey.

Members of my extended support team—Art Turock. Alison Miller, and Anton Kowalski—thanks for pushing and shoving me toward success. Sabrina Zaslov, my nutrition advisor—thank you for your great commonsense advice. Dr. Lee Rice, my personal physician—you have always been there when I needed you and I am grateful. Members of my men's group, particularly Dene Oliver—you helped me realize that the real motivation had to come from me. Dan Epstein—thank you for being my prostate buddy and constant truth teller. Mike Ortmeier—you are a servant leader extraordinaire. Thank you for constantly helping me keep my commitment to my commitment.

Members of my Blanchard support team—Margery Allen, Anna Espino, and Martha Lawrence—you are always there to cheer me on and point me in the right direction. Renee Broadwell, you are not only an important member of my Blanchard team but also Tim's and my partner on this book. Thanks for working side by side with us and helping us massage every word and phrase.

Tim Kearin

Since this book is the project of a lifetime for me, I have many to thank and acknowledge.

Most important, I want to thank my coauthor and great friend, Ken Blanchard. Without your dedication, hard work, and mentorship, this book would not be possible. Renee Broadwell, as editor you have masterfully transformed my ideas into script and supported me so well on this project. I also wish to thank Martha Lawrence, executive editor for The Ken Blanchard Companies, for standing by me and encouraging me during the early stages of the book formulation. And Dr. Nick Yphantides, author of *My Big Fat Greek Diet*, I thank you for your advice and coaching on the book.

My wife Sharon, life and business partner for so many years, I thank you for your encouragement and support in helping me with ideas and editing throughout this entire three-year project. To my son Deyl and his wife Paige, and to my daughter Kasey and her husband Skye, thanks for the encouragement and for always being there.

Finally, Ken and Tim would both like to thank Steve Piersanti of Berrett-Koehler Publishers along with his fabulous team: Charlotte Ashlock, Courtney Shonfeld, David Marshall, Dianne Platner, Jeevan Sivasubramaniam, Kat Engh, Katie Sheehan, Kristen Frantz, Kylah Frazier, Marina Cook, Michael Crowley, Neal Maillet, Rick Wilson, and Zoe Mackey, as well as the good folks at Michael Bass Associates. They are all exceptional partners.

Index

About the Authors

Ken Blanchard

Few people have impacted the day-to-day management of people and companies more than Ken Blanchard. A gregarious and sought-after author, speaker, and business consultant, Ken is universally characterized as one of the most insightful, powerful, and compassionate individuals in business today.

From his phenomenal best-selling book *The One Minute Manager* (coauthored with Spencer Johnson)—which has sold more than 15 million copies and has remained on best-seller lists for more than 25 years—to the library of books including *Raving Fans, Gung Ho!, Leadership and the One Minute Manager, Whale Done!*, and many others he has coauthored with outstanding practitioners—Ken's impact as a writer is far-reaching. In July 2005, he was inducted into the Amazon Hall of Fame as one of the top 25 best-selling authors of all time.

Ken is the chief spiritual officer of The Ken Blanchard Companies, an international management training and consulting firm that he and his wife, Dr. Marjorie Blanchard, founded in 1979 in San Diego. He is a visiting lecturer at his alma mater, Cornell University, where he is a trustee emeritus of the board of trustees. Ken is also cofounder of Lead Like Jesus, a nonprofit organization.

Ken and Margie have been married 51 years and live in San Diego. Their son Scott, their daughter Debbie, and Scott's wife Madeleine all hold key positions at The Ken Blanchard Companies.

Tim Kearin

Tim Kearin has been in the health and fitness industry for more than 40 years. His interest in strength training helped him become a standout high school athlete and took him to the University of Arizona on an athletic scholarship. After graduation, Tim began a career as an army officer, where his fitness expertise led to a graduate degree from Indiana University and a subsequent assignment to the physical education department at the United States Military Academy. Army's new football coach at the time, NFL coaching legend Lou Saban, recognized Tim's talents and made him the team's strength and conditioning coach, a position Tim held for six years. In 1984, Tim expanded his fitness résumé by becoming the fitness director at the Hughston Clinic in Columbus, Georgia.

In 1986, Tim and his wife Sharon moved to San Diego, California, and founded Personally Fit, Inc., a health and fitness company focused on adult fitness, specialized personal training, and physical therapy. After 20 years, Tim sold the business to pursue other specialized interests, including the work he did with Ken Blanchard that became the basis for this book.

Tim and Sharon, a dancer and fitness practitioner, have been married 36 years and live in San Diego. Their son Deyl and daughter Kasey live in Santa Barbara with their families and are fitness enthusiasts as well.

Services Available

The Ken Blanchard Companies®

The Ken Blanchard Companies is a global leader in workplace learning, productivity, performance, and leadership effectiveness that is best known for its Situational Leadership® II program—the most widely taught leadership model in the world. Because of its ability to help people excel as self-leaders and leaders of others, SLII® is embraced by Fortune 500 companies as well as small to midsize businesses, governments, and educational and nonprofit organizations.

Blanchard® programs, which are based on the evidence that people are the key to accomplishing strategic objectives and driving business results, develop excellence in leadership, teams, customer loyalty, change management, and performance improvement. The company's continual research points to best practices for workplace improvement, while its world-class trainers and coaches drive organizational and behavioral change at all levels and help people make the shift from learning to doing.

Leadership experts from The Ken Blanchard Companies are available for workshops and consulting as well as keynote addresses on organizational development, workplace

performance, and business trends. Visit kenblanchard.com
to learn about workshops, coaching services, and leadership
programs to help your organization create lasting behavior
changes that have a measurable impact.

The Ken Blanchard Companies
World Headquarters
125 State Place
Escondido, California 92029
United States
+1-760-489-5005
International@kenblanchard.com
www.kenblanchard.com

United Kingdom
The Ken Blanchard Companies UK
+44 (0) 1483 456300
uk@kenblanchard.com
www.kenblanchard.com/E-mail/?vlc=28

Canada
The Ken Blanchard Companies Canada
+1 905 829-3510
Canada@kenblanchard.com
www.kenblanchard.com/E-mail/?vlc=5

Singapore
The Ken Blanchard Companies Singapore
+65-6775 1030
Singapore@kenblanchard.com
www.kenblanchard.com/contact/?vlc=200

Australia
Blanchard International Australia
+61 2 9858 2822
Australia@kenblanchard.com
www.blanchardinternational.com.au

India
Blanchard International India
+91-124-4511970
India@kenblanchard.com
www.blanchardinternational.co.in

Ireland
Blanchard International Ireland
+353 879614320
Ireland@kenblanchard.com
www.blanchardinternational.ie

New Zealand
Blanchard International New Zealand
+64 (0) 27 510 5009 / 0800 25 26 24
newzealand@kenblanchard.com
www.blanchard.co.nz

Join Us Online

Visit Blanchard on YouTube
Watch thought leaders from The Ken Blanchard Companies in action. Link and subscribe to Ken Blanchard's channel and you'll receive updates as new videos are posted.

Join the Blanchard Fan Club on Facebook
Be part of our inner circle and link to Ken Blanchard on Facebook. Meet other fans of Ken and his books, access videos and photos, and get invited to special events.

Join Conversations with Ken Blanchard
Ken Blanchard's blog, HowWeLead.org, was created to inspire positive change. It is a public service site devoted to leadership topics that connect us all, a social network where you will meet people who care deeply about responsible leadership, and a place where Ken would like to hear your opinion.

Ken's Twitter Updates
Receive timely messages and thoughts from Ken. Find out the events he's attending and what's on his mind @ kenblanchard.

How2Lead App
The free How2Lead app allows you to stay up-to-date with the latest in leadership, corporate training, and management practices. Read Blanchard blogs, access videos, and receive updates on new thought leadership and research. Compatible with Android phones and devices, iPhone, iPod touch, and iPad.

Tim Kearin

Fit at Last by Design is a health and fitness company owned and operated by Tim Kearin. Tim has been working in the health and fitness industry for more than 40 years as a strength and conditioning coach, a specialized personal trainer for all age levels, a fitness and physical therapy facility owner and operator, a clinical consultant, and an author.

Services include consulting in the above-mentioned disciplines, corporate fitness development, keynote addresses, workshops, comprehensive fitness evaluations, and coaching services. Visit Fitatlastbydesign.com to learn about ways that you and your organization can develop and sustain a greater level of health and wellness.

Contact:

Fit at Last by Design, Inc.
P.O. Box 27720
San Diego, CA 92198

866-348-2852 toll-free

Fitatlastbydesign.com

Also by Ken Blanchard

Ken Blanchard and Mark Miller

Great Leaders Grow
Becoming a Leader for Life

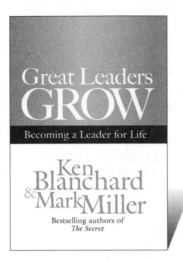

What is the secret to lasting as a leader? As Ken Blanchard and Mark Miller write, "The path to increased influence, impact, and leadership effectiveness is paved with personal growth...Our capacity to grow determines our capacity to lead." In *Great Leaders Grow*, Debbie Brewster becomes a mentor to Blake, her own mentor's young son. She tells him: "How well you and I serve will be determined by the decision to grow or not. Will you be a leader who is always ready to face the next challenge? Or will you be a leader who tries to apply yesterday's solutions to today's problems?" As Debbie leads Blake through the four growth areas that every leader must focus on, you'll be inspired to make your own long-term plan for professional and personal growth.

Hardcover, 144 pages, ISBN 978-1-60994-303-5
PDF ebook, ISBN 978-1-60509-695-7

BK Berrett–Koehler Publishers, Inc.
San Francisco, *www.bkconnection.com*   **800.929.2929**

Ken Blanchard and Mark Miller

The Secret
What Great Leaders Know and Do, Second Edition

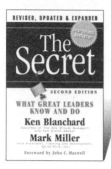

Join struggling young executive Debbie Brewster as she explores a profound yet seemingly contradictory concept: to lead is to serve. Along the way she learns why great leaders seem preoccupied with the future, what three arenas require continuous improvement, the two essential components of leadership success, how to knowingly strengthen—or unwittingly destroy—leadership credibility, and more.

Hardcover, 144 pages, ISBN 978-1-60509-268-3
PDF ebook, ISBN 978-1-60509-470-0

Ken Blanchard and Jesse Lyn Stoner

Full Steam Ahead!
Unleash the Power of Vision in Your Work and Your Life

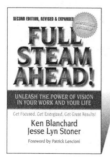

The lessons of *Full Steam Ahead!* are revealed through the inspirational story of two people who create an inspiring vision for the place they work and for their own lives. Together they discover the three elements of a compelling vision: a significant purpose, clear values, and a picture of the future. By understanding how a vision is created, communicated, and lived, they discover how to make that vision come alive.

Hardcover, 216 pages, ISBN 978-1-60509-875-3
PDF ebook, ISBN 978-1-60509-876-0

BK® Berrett–Koehler Publishers, Inc.
San Francisco, *www.bkconnection.com*   **800.929.2929**

Berrett–Koehler
BK̄ Publishers

A community dedicated to creating
a world that works for all

Dear Reader,

Thank you for picking up this book and joining our worldwide community of Berrett-Koehler readers. We share ideas that bring positive change into people's lives, organizations, and society.

To welcome you, we'd like to offer you a free e-book. You can pick from among twelve of our bestselling books by entering the promotional code **BKP92E** here: http://www.bkconnection.com/welcome.

When you claim your free e-book, we'll also send you a copy of our e-newsletter, the *BK Communiqué*. Although you're free to unsubscribe, there are many benefits to sticking around. In every issue of our newsletter you'll find

- A free e-book
- Tips from famous authors
- Discounts on spotlight titles
- Hilarious insider publishing news
- A chance to win a prize for answering a riddle

Best of all, our readers tell us, "Your newsletter is the only one I actually read." So claim your gift today, and please stay in touch!

Sincerely,

Charlotte Ashlock
Steward of the BK Website

Questions? Comments? Contact me at bkcommunity@bkpub.com.

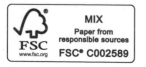

Situational Leadership® II Model

Leadership Styles

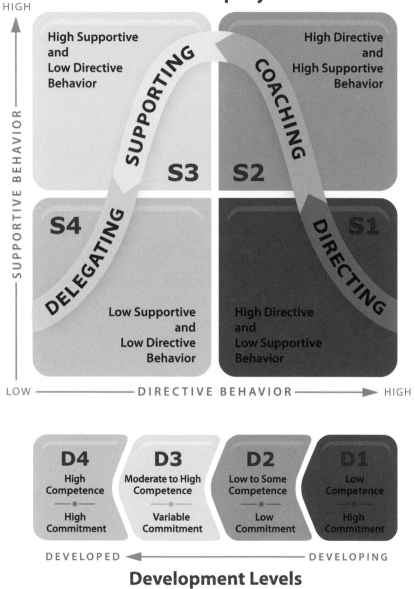